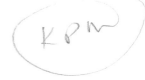
The Good Appraisal
Toolkit for Primary Care

Ruth Chambers
General Practitioner
Clinical Dean
Staffordshire University
Head of Stoke-on-Trent Teaching PCT Programme

Abdol Tavabie
General Practitioner
GP Dean (Director of Postgraduate General Practice Education)
Kent, Surrey and Sussex Deanery
Vice-Chair of COGPED

Kay Mohanna
General Practitioner
Principal Lecturer in Medical Education
Staffordshire University
Lead for GP Appraisal
West Midlands Deanery

and

Gill Wakley
Freelance General Practitioner
Visiting Professor
Centre for Health Policy and Practice
Staffordshire University

Radcliffe Publishing
Oxford • San Francisco

Radcliffe Publishing Ltd
18 Marcham Road
Abingdon
Oxon OX14 1AA
United Kingdom

www.radcliffe-oxford.com
Electronic catalogue and worldwide online ordering facility.

British Library Cataloguing in Publication Data

A catalogue record for this book is available from the British Library.

ISBN 1 85775 602 9

A 041614

W 89

Typeset by Advance Typesetting Ltd, Oxfordshire
Printed and bound by TJ International Ltd, Padstow, Cornwall

Contents

Preface   vii

About the authors   ix

Acknowledgements   xi

Chapter 1: Introduction   1
    Definitions and context   1
    Appraisal, assessment and evaluation   2
    Implementing appraisal as an effective process in trusts: 3
      roles and responsibilities of primary care organisations
    Organisational commitment to appraisal   4
    Implementing effective appraisal   6
    Quality assurance   8
    Context of appraisal and revalidation for doctors   9
    Appraisal and professional regulation for healthcare professions 10
    Education, training and appraisal indicators in the new 11
      general medical services contract

Chapter 2: Making the most of your appraisal: 13
when being appraised
    Linking your personal development plan to appraisal   14
    Ten examples of tools and techniques to provide evidence 19
      of your performance at work for your appraisal portfolio
    Professional development activities to help you be a more 24
      effective learner or professional
    Preparing for your appraisal   35

Chapter 3: Being an effective appraiser   41
    Preparing for the appraisal session as an appraiser   42
    Timetable for the appraisal process: countdown as an appraiser 43
    Pitfalls in appraisal   45
    Ground rules   47
    Qualities of an appraiser   49
    Distinguish the appraiser role from others you might have 50
    Anticipating and overcoming likely barriers in the   51
      appraisal discussion

Chapter 4:   Developing your competence as an appraiser in   57
communication skills and encouraging others in their
professional development
    Setting out your knowledge and skills as an appraiser based   57
       on the NHS Knowledge and Skills Framework
    Dimension 1. Communication: consistently practise good   60
       communication skills (Level 4)
    Dimension 2. Personal and people development: develop own   76
       and others' knowledge and practice across professional and
       organisational boundaries in relation to appraisal (Level 5)
    Reflect on your own personal development or that of those   78
       you appraise

Chapter 5:   Developing your competence as an appraiser in   87
enabling others to perform well and improve their delivery
of healthcare
    Dimension 3. Health, safety and security: promote others'   87
       health, safety and security in relation to appraisal (Level 1)
    Dimension 4. Service development: contribute to development   92
       of services (i.e. services for patients and the appraisal process)
       (Level 3)
    Dimension 5. Quality improvement: demonstrate personal   96
       commitment to quality improvement, offering others advice
       and support as an integral part of appraisal process (Level 4)
    Dimension 6. Equality, diversity and rights: enable others to   99
       exercise their rights and promote equal opportunities and
       diversity through appraisal (Level 4)
    Dimension 7. Promotion of self-care and peer support: 101
       encourage others to promote their own health and wellbeing
       through the appraisal process (Level 1)
    Dimension 8. Ability to manage the appraisal process: 104
       process and manage data and information and maintain
       confidentiality (Level 3)
    Dimension 9. Ability to carry out needs assessment: 108
       interpret, analyse and synthesise data and information
       appropriately, within appraisal process (Level 3)
    Dimension 10. Ability to contribute to and/or co-ordinate the   111
       support system for the appraisal process: develop and sustain
       partnership working with those appraised and the practice/
       PCO/Deanery (as appropriate) (appraiser Level 2; appraiser
       lead Level 4)

Dimension 11. Leadership skills: lead others in the development   114
    of knowledge, ideas and work practice as an integral part of the
    appraisal process (Level 2)
And lastly ... protected time: identify and negotiate protected   117
    time to devote to the appraisal process

Chapter 6:   Demonstrating your competence as an appraiser   119
    Five stages in organising your evidence   119
    Collecting data to demonstrate your learning, competence and   123
        performance as an appraiser

Chapter 7:   Linking appraisal with career planning, career   131
development and career enhancement
    Your career review   131
    Factors to consider in *reviewing* or *choosing* a career specialty   132
        or interest
    Job evaluation   133
    Job satisfaction and career fulfilment   134
    Appreciating your personal ethics and work values   134
    Motivation   135
    Relationship between continuing professional development   135
        and career development
    Consider finding a mentor   143

Chapter 8:   Evaluation and assessment of appraisal   145
    Thinking about evaluation and assessment of the appraisal   145
        process
    The evaluation cycle: outcomes of appraisal   146
    Evaluation questions   147
    Participant evaluation: appraiser and individuals who have   148
        been appraised
    Ideas for evaluating the appraiser   155
    Peer review   156
    Primary care organisation, or trust, or Deanery perspective   159
    Patient perspective   163
    Conclusions   163

Chapter 9:   Being an effective primary care organisation: 167
using appraisal as a tool for continuing improvement
    Resources necessary for effective appraisal   167
    Systems and processes necessary within organisations for   169
        effective appraisal
    Setting up a quality assurance framework for appraisal   171
    Summary   174

Appendix 1   **Template for a job description and person**   175
                 specification of an appraiser, based on the NHS
                 Knowledge and Skills Framework
Appendix 2   **Example of a template for your personal**   178
                 professional development plan – start with one
                 main topic and build others on as you justify
                 needing to learn more about them
Appendix 3   **Structured review of the quality of the personal**   182
                 development plan
Appendix 4   **Example of an honorary contract for**   185
                 independent contractor (e.g. GP, dentist,
                 pharmacist, optometrist) acting as appraiser
                 for a primary care organisation: statement of
                 terms and conditions
Appendix 5   **Sources of help in relation to appraisal**   188

Index   191

Preface

We are pleased to welcome you to this toolkit, which has grown out of our work at the Kent, Surrey and Sussex (KSS) GP Deanery over the past two years.

In 2001, the KSS GP Deanery submitted a strategic proposal for workforce development within the primary care setting. The proposal had the full support of the KSS Workforce Development Confederation for funding to support a network of primary care staff. We invited each primary care trust (PCT) to appoint a full-time primary care workforce tutor to work closely with GP tutors in supporting *all* members of primary care in their personal development and appraisal processes. This unique approach to lifelong learning has created opportunities for everyone's development through the appraisal process.

The KSS GP Deanery appointed three lifelong learning advisors as project managers to join the GP Deanery to support and promote multiprofessional working and learning. The lifelong learning advisors work closely with the locality associate GP deans and act as a conduit between the GP Deanery and PCTs. Their contribution and support in the GP Deanery modernisation agenda have been rich and highly welcome.

The emphasis of the work of both lifelong learning advisors and primary care workforce tutors alongside their GP colleagues has been:

- promotion of teamwork across professional and organisational boundaries
- maximising the contribution of all staff to patient care through the appraisal process
- ensuring that all staff are equipped with the skills they need to work in a complex, changing NHS
- developing new, more flexible careers for all
- creating a responsive learning environment
- reviewing and planning the redesign of the workforce to meet the current and the future demands in the NHS.

The KSS GP Deanery has been increasingly involved with the GP NHS appraisal process in initial training of appraisers and setting up continuing support for them at the local level. We also recognised the importance of defining the competency of appraisers so that it is aligned with the NHS Competency Framework. This work was led by Professor Ruth Chambers, who, with the help of her colleagues, defined the job description and person specifications of appraisers.

We have experimented with a number of ideas in our regular joint conferences with GP and primary care workforce tutors, developing their skills in facilitation and negotiating their multiprofessional agenda at the local level. It has become clear that, in order to promote an appraisal process in primary care, and in particular in general practice, we need an appraisal toolkit. Our goal was to develop a toolkit that allows the individual and organisation's (such as practice, PCT or Deanery) appraiser to appreciate the process, which should clearly be traced back to their development and ultimately improve patient care. This is very important in the implementation of the new general medical services (GMS) and personal medical services (PMS) contracts in general practice.

This toolkit has been prepared in response to this agenda and requests from our workforce. It is not a cookbook, but offers routes to support each individual and his or her organisation in the promotion of quality patient care through encouraging individual development. It is generalisable to all primary care settings. The toolkit will help you to implement good practice in appraisal whether you are an individual health professional or manager appraising others or being appraised yourself, within a practice (general medical, pharmacy, optometry or dental) or clinical discipline (medical, nursing, allied health professions) and/or employed by a primary care organisation (PCO) – anywhere in the UK. The toolkit will be instrumental to you and your organisation realising the benefits of appraisal in encouraging staff development and improved delivery of patient care.

We are grateful to all those who have contributed and commented on the evolution of the appraisal process and acted as test beds for the future.

Professor Abdol Tavabie
August 2004

About the authors

Ruth Chambers has been a GP for more than 20 years. Her previous experience has encompassed a wide range of research and educational activities, including stress and the health of doctors, the quality of healthcare, healthy working, teenagers' contraception and many other topics.

She is currently a part-time GP, Head of Stoke-on-Trent Teaching Primary Care Trust programme and the Professor of Primary Care Development at the Faculty of Health and Sciences at Staffordshire University. She was the Chair of Staffordshire Medical Audit Advisory Group and a GP trainer for four years. Ruth has initiated and run all types of educational initiatives and activities, including appraiser training workshops.

Abdol Tavabie has been a GP for the past 20 years. His practice in Orpington, Kent, was the second practice in the country to achieve BS5750 for clinical and organisational standards, in 1991. Abdol has been involved in GP education in various posts over the years, including being GP trainer, VTS course organiser and chairman of a Medical Audit Advisory Group. He is now GP Dean (Director of Postgraduate General Practice Education) for Kent, Surrey and Sussex Deanery, and Vice-Chair of COGPED (Committee of General Practice Education Directors). He is also Professor of Primary Care at the School of Health, Brighton University.

Kay Mohanna is a principal in general practice, a GP trainer and Principal Lecturer in Medical Education at Staffordshire University. She is responsible for development and delivery of the Masters in Medical Education, and is lead tutor for the ethics module of the Masters in Primary Care. She has developed and run *Teaching the Teachers* courses for consultants, dentists, GPs, physiotherapists, cytologists and other health professional groups, and is co-facilitator on the West Midlands modular GP trainers course.

Kay is the West Midlands Deanery lead for GP appraisal. She runs the Deanery appraisal support programme, organised the 2003 regional conference on Appraisal and edited *Appraisal for GPs*, a supplement to the journal *Education for Primary Care* (Radcliffe Medical Press, 2003).

Gill Wakley started in general practice but transferred to community medicine shortly afterwards, and then moved into public health. A desire for increased contact with patients caused a move back into general practice. She has been heavily involved in learning and teaching throughout her career. She worked in a training general practice and was a senior clinical lecturer with the Primary Care Department at Keele University. Like Ruth, she has run all types of educational initiatives and activities, including training GP appraisers. A visiting professor at Staffordshire University, she now works as a freelance GP, writer and lecturer, including co-authoring another related book, *Appraisal for the Apprehensive* (Radcliffe Medical Press, 2002), with Ruth.

Contributor

Wendy Garcarz is an education and development specialist with a proven record of accomplishment in primary care. She has 20 years' experience in education and training management in both the public and private sectors. She has spent the past 10 years working in primary care, developing primary care clinicians and support workers in service commissioning, continuing professional development, strategic planning and service innovations.

Wendy is the Chief Executive of *4 health*, an organisational development consultancy specialising in sustainable change through workforce investment. She and her colleagues work with all types of healthcare organisations (wendy@4-health.biz).

Acknowledgements

We have drawn on much of our recent work in continuing education and appraisal in compiling this *Good Appraisal Toolkit*. In particular, we have extracted substantial material from related works co-authored by Ruth, Kay and Gill. Wendy Garcarz wrote most of Chapter 1 for this book. Some of our material has been derived from developmental work in appraisal in our respective Deaneries; in Kent, Surrey and Sussex, where Abdol and colleagues have led on appraisal for all members of primary care teams; and the West Midlands, where Dr Stephen Kelly, Director of GP Postgraduate Education, has enabled the Midland Faculty of the Royal College of General Practitioners to train, develop and support GP appraisers. We are grateful to Stephen Kelly for allowing us to reproduce evaluation and process tools for appraisal produced within the Deanery.

1

Introduction

Definitions and context

A definition of appraisal that encapsulates the developmental purpose of appraisal is 'a professional process of constructive dialogue in which the [person] being appraised has a formal structured opportunity to reflect on his or her work and to consider how his or her effectiveness might be improved'.[1] The drive to introduce formal appraisals came initially as part of the programme to introduce clinical governance across the NHS, as laid out in the 1998 consultation document *A First Class Service*.[2]

Appraisal is widely accepted in the NHS as a formative process that should be concerned with the professional development and personal fulfilment of the individual, leading to an improvement in their performance at work. This positive interpretation of the appraisal process supports the delivery of high-quality patient care and drive to improve clinical standards. Appraisal has been in place in industry, commerce and the public sector for decades. In the NHS, health professionals, managers and administrative staff are now all expected to undergo annual appraisals. In England, appraisal became a contractual requirement for all hospital consultants from April 2001 and all GP principals and personal medical services (PMS) equivalent doctors from April 2002, as part of their forthcoming revalidation system.

In addition to the NHS expectations that nurses will have an annual appraisal, the Nursing and Midwifery Council (NMC) requires nurses to maintain a professional portfolio (www.nmc-uk.org). The onus is on individual nurses to decide how they will collect and keep the information that will demonstrate to the NMC that they are clinically competent and that they have taken on board the concept of lifelong learning. Nurses themselves need to decide the nature of the information they collect and retain in their portfolio to reflect their everyday roles and responsibilities. Nurses have been engaged in portfolio demonstration of their learning activity through their PREP (post-registration education and practice) requirements since 1995.[3] All community nurses – district nurses, health visitors and practice nurses – should receive appraisal and clinical supervision as part of that PREP process.

In the NHS, the appraiser is usually the line manager – except for independent contractors (GPs, pharmacists, dentists, optometrists) who do not have a 'line manager', in which case a CPD tutor, colleague or peer may be appointed as their appraiser. It is good practice to allow the person being appraised to opt for an alternative person to be their appraiser other than their line manager, if there are sensitive issues to discuss that affect the line manager.

Appraisal, assessment and evaluation

There is confusion relating to the terms 'appraisal', 'assessment' and 'evaluation'. The Department of Health differentiated between appraisal and assessment in its 1990s vision for the widespread uptake of appraisal (*see* Box 1.1).[4]

Box 1.1: Differentiating between appraisal and assessment[4]

Appraisal is a positive process to give someone feedback on their performance, to chart their continuing progress and to identify development needs. It is a forward-looking process essential for the developmental and educational planning needs of an individual.

Assessment is the process of measuring progress against agreed criteria ... It is not the primary aim of appraisal to scrutinise doctors to see if they are performing poorly, but rather to help them consolidate and improve on good performance aiming towards excellence.

Assessment and appraisal both concern the individual. Assessment, in educational terms, implies a 'judgement' being made about the individual and is defined as the process of measuring an individual's progress against pre-defined quality standards and criteria. However, assessment can also mean the process of identifying the presence or absence of learning arising from an educational event, when assessment is a judgement about the extent to which educational objectives have been attained by the individual. Within the context of general practice training, assessment has been separated into two components, summative and formative assessment. The former relates to the achieving of set standards at an end point (pass/fail) and the latter term relates to the educational development of the individual learner.[5]

There is a subtle difference between appraisal and formative assessment, as emphasised in Box 1.1. Appraisal, as already stated, is a process whereby, through constructive and regular dialogue, feedback on performance in relation to personal goals, and assistance in progression towards those goals is given. Within the definition of appraisal there is an acceptance that while there may be general criteria, the process allows for the individual learner to determine his or her own standing and create relevant goals. In appraisal, the main focus is the learner's estimation of his or her own performance in relation to goals he or she has determined, whereas formative assessment examines progress in respect of jointly agreed learning objectives with the teacher giving feedback in relation to these goals. These learning objectives have an element of personal choice but are nevertheless constrained by the need to deliver health services within the NHS.[6-9]

Evaluation concerns the teacher and is an attempt to identify and interpret the effectiveness of teaching and associated programmes.[6] Within the field of education there are many different approaches and philosophies that can be employed. These vary from the teacher-centred approach, which seeks to evaluate a teaching intervention only in terms of whether pre-determined objectives have been met, to participatory evaluation, which seeks to actively include the learners in evaluating the whole of the teaching (*see* Chapter 8 for more in-depth consideration of evaluation). One model of evaluation that would appear easily accessible is Kirkpatrick's hierarchy.[10]

Here, evaluation can be considered in terms of learner satisfaction, acquisition of skills or knowledge, change in behaviour and impact on the wider society.

Although evaluation is generally deemed necessary and important, it is seldom implemented.

Implementing appraisal as an effective process in trusts: roles and responsibilities of primary care organisations

With the current change agenda in the NHS involving the restructuring and redefining of roles and responsibilities of organisations and individuals, the government is keen to show the validity and effectiveness of the modernisation agenda. Organisational developments are expected to:

- promote the objectives and outcomes of organisations
- show real benefits in terms of achieving national targets and local priorities
- provide strong and effective leadership
- build public confidence in the NHS.

A key strand of modernisation of the NHS is performance management, on both an organisational and individual basis. It is now recognised that performance management through staff appraisal brings significant benefits when conducted in a learning environment, as it is one of the few managerial theories and techniques that can produce sustainable change without adversely affecting retention and morale of staff.

The development of a learning culture is a practical measure to enable the workforce to regularly hone their skills and knowledge and deliver their primary care organisation's (PCO) objectives through quality care services. A foundation stone of the learning culture is a systematic and effective appraisal scheme that links the organisational objectives with the professional and personal objectives of its staff. It also provides another demonstration of the organisation's commitment to the continued renewal of its intellectual capital.

The process has many names – such as individual performance review (IPR), staff appraisal and development needs review (DNR) – but most organisations view appraisal as a mechanism for reviewing past performance. However, to use it purely for that purpose is to ignore significant organisational and individual benefits that effective appraisals can deliver, consolidating continuing professional development and validating clinical competence. While details vary from profession to profession the educational principles remain the same.

The aims of an effective appraisal scheme are:

- to give individuals feedback on their performance
- to explore the limits of their current knowledge and skills
- to offer a systematic development needs analysis process for all members of staff
- to produce personal development plans that establish how training and development needs will be met
- to disseminate corporate objectives throughout the workforce
- to establish individual objectives enabling staff members to understand their contribution.

The aims of one primary care trust's (PCT) appraisal process, given in Box 1.2, reflects this approach.[11]

Box 1.2:   Long-term aims of employee appraisal in North Stoke Teaching Primary Care Trust[11]

- To help you make the most of yourself
- To help the PCT make the most effective use of its employees

The role of the manager/appraiser is to fit the two aims together.

   Employee appraisal is:

- an opportunity to stimulate you through praise and encouragement
- a chance to reflect
- a chance to discuss any problem areas
- a brainstorming session on your working relationships
- a chance to consider your future career plans
- the opportunity to identify and plan training and development needs and opportunities.

   Employee appraisal is *not*:

- a substitute for disciplinary procedure
- an opportunity to list all your gripes from the previous year
- an opportunity to belittle a member of staff or put them in their place
- a chance for a manager/appraiser to tell a member of staff what they need to do for the next 12 months.

An appraisal provides a mechanism for identifying training needs from both the individual's and the organisation's perspectives. There should be a balance between both in order to reflect the need to achieve national targets and the workforce's learning aspirations. An effective feedback system from individual appraisals can identify and anticipate skills gaps across the PCO.

The model in Figure 1.1 describes a simple corporate planning framework that illustrates the importance of effective appraisals feeding into the processes of performance management, workforce planning and change management in the trust.

Organisational commitment to appraisal

The PCO's commitment to appraisal needs to be a central strand of its human resource, service quality, performance management, and training and development strategies. It links these key areas together.

The drivers for healthcare organisations are focused around their performance. Clinical performance is verified through clinical effectiveness, governance and risk management. Financial performance is measured in relation to income and expenditure balance, robust audit methods and consistency. Operational performance is measured by recruitment and retention of skilled staff, the ability to maintain skill and knowledge bases, and efficient performance of staff and other resources. The effectiveness of

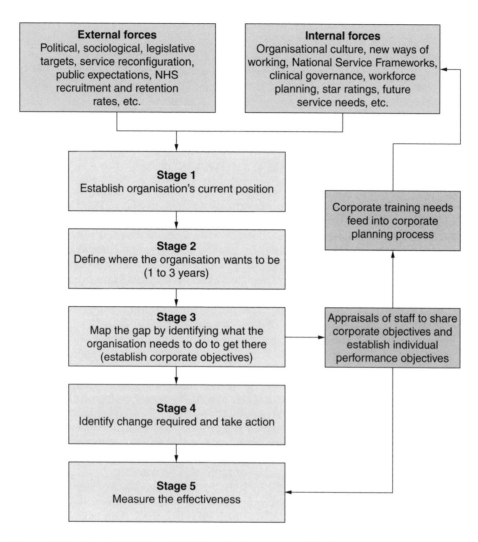

Figure 1.1: Appraisals integrated into a simple corporate planning process in a trust.

such organisational mechanisms rests on the capability, competence and motivation of its workforce to deliver against pre-determined performance objectives.

Appraisal is the most effective mechanism an organisation can deploy to focus the workforce on its objectives. As a key element in a performance management strategy, organisations need to display genuine commitment to the process. They need to invest in it, promote it and use sanctions against those who would ignore it.

The commitment usually manifests itself in expectations that everyone will undergo an appraisal annually, and the information gathered about training and educational needs is used to design and commission training for the following year. Innovative organisations take this a stage further by using the information to feed into corporate and strategy planning, shaping future services, role redesign and service reconfiguration.

From an individual's perspective, it is important that the appraisal process includes a half-year review. The constantly changing environment of the NHS means that any objectives (organisational or individual) set at the initial appraisal meeting are likely to alter during the following year. The organisation may need to adapt strategies and initiatives during that year to ensure flexibility, and that effort is focused in the right areas. A mid-year review provides an effective mechanism for that type of change management to take place with the workforce.

Implementing effective appraisal

An organisation launching an appraisal process needs to make preparations to ensure that the workforce understands the importance and potential benefits of appraisal to them as individuals, as much as to their organisation. The overall design of the scheme should have very clear objectives in terms of what it can deliver to the organisation, and clear benefits to the individual. The workforce will receive any organisational change with a certain amount of anxiety or cynicism, but the introduction of an appraisal scheme may heighten the response as any type of performance monitoring is a sensitive and emotive issue. The organisational climate will dictate the response to a certain degree, but those responsible for implementation should be sensitive to the messages given out and work hard to promote the positive benefits of appraisal.

Some organisations spend significant time and money developing the paperwork systems that underpin the process. There are huge resources freely available on the Internet and in workbooks that can be adapted to any organisational requirements, within and outside the health sector (www.appraisaluk.info, www.dh.gov.uk/PolicyAnd Guidance/HumanResourcesAndTraining/LearningAndPersonalDevelopment/Appraisals/ fs/en and www.businessballs.com). There is little to choose between content, although styles vary considerably, and the simpler the process the easier the appraisal system will be to manage. The paperwork is incidental compared with the appraisal experience itself, which should be a professionally conducted discussion that moves the participants forward, and as a result drives the organisation forward too.

The standard of appraisal should be high and the organisation should be open about its expectations of best practice in this area. If the workforce sense that the organisation views appraisal as a 'tick-box exercise' then their commitment to the process will be half-hearted and little benefit will be gained by going through the motions of staff appraisal.

Promoting the benefits of appraisal is an essential part of the process and should be done throughout the planning, design and implementation of an appraisal scheme. It is not a one-off activity, but something that should be done regularly and systematically to ensure that everyone in the organisation is exposed to the positive benefits of appraisal. The good practice in appraisal that has been established in KSS Deanery for all primary care team members (*see* Preface) is reflected in the Committee of General Practice Education Directors' (COGPED) recommendations (*see* Box 1.3).

Training is essential to ensure that both appraisers and those appraised understand what is expected and that they have the skills and understanding to make it an effective process. In organisations where effective appraisal is recognised as a significant contributor to organisational performance, appraisal training is included as part of mandatory training, with updates and competence checks done on a three-yearly basis. It is usual in NHS organisations for appraisal to be seen as an integral part of a line manager's role. However, it is naive to assume that all line managers have the

---

Box 1.3: COGPED recommendations for the roles and responsibilities for Deaneries[12]

The roles and responsibilities of the Deanery and of their GP tutors need to be defined and appropriately supported. In particular Deaneries need to:

1 support the process of appraisal and the training of appraisers
2 align GP tutors with PCOs and adjust their role away from 'signing off' personal development plans (PDPs) towards supporting continuing professional development (CPD) more broadly
3 ensure that appraisers accredit (sign off) PDPs satisfactorily
4 ensure that GP registrars are prepared for annual appraisal on graduation
5 support and develop appraisers
6 oversee the content of appraisal
7 ensure appraisal outcomes.

In KSS Deanery this includes:

- the recruitment and training of GP appraisers
- training and ongoing professional support of GP appraisers (learning sets for GP and other professional appraisers)
- liaison by appraisers with CPD providers and PCTs in meeting learning needs identified through the appraisal process.

---

right knowledge, skill and competence required to conduct appraisals. The skills required are often viewed as those of generic communication, but there are complex dynamics at play when an individual's ability to do his or her job well is under scrutiny.

Giving and receiving constructive feedback, setting performance goals and human motivational theory are three key factors in appraisers delivering effective appraisals that are not yet a routine in the NHS. If a PCO is to gain any benefit from conducting appraisals it needs to invest in the skills and competencies that make it an effective process.

Integrating the needs of different professions into an appraisal scheme is important to ensure that it accommodates all requirements and does not require parallel processes or activities. Professional portfolio development may run alongside an appraisal scheme and support the process. Duplication of the portfolio for other purposes should be eradicated as staff would use it as an excuse for non-participation. It is important for the process to be perceived by all elements of the workforce as a fair and equitable process, and not just an activity reserved for those with qualifications.

Consistency of application gives a strong message to the whole organisation that performance quality is something expected from all, not just those directly involved in delivering patient care. Large organisations may need to phase in the introduction of an appraisal scheme due to simple logistics of training. In such cases, it is wise to publish the complete implementation timetable so that all levels of staff see where they fit into the process. That phased implementation should have given some consideration to the penalties of non-compliance with the appraisal scheme. If the organisational policy states that everyone has to undergo an annual appraisal with a mid-term review, how is that being measured? Very few schemes have any monitoring data available, and if checks are made, it tends to be about whether an appraisal took place, rather than how effective it was. This approach is reflected by the staff surveys conducted recently in NHS trusts as part of the Improving Working Lives (IWL) assessments.[13] Anecdotal evidence puts average rates of appraisals received between 65 and 80% (the figure is even less for mid-term reviews), and yet if it is an organisational priority why are organisations not recording 100% take-up rates?

There are few meaningful monitors and no sanctions for managers who fail to conduct annual appraisals. The picture is that most PCOs can find pockets of good practice where appraisal and mid-term reviews are done very effectively and are reaping benefits for individuals, teams and the wider organisation. The key success factors in effective appraisal schemes are:

- consistency of application
- competence of the appraiser
- quality of the appraisal interview from the viewpoints of those appraised.

Even when an appraisal scheme has been in operation for a while, PCOs need to have a monitoring process in place to quality assure appraisal interviews and how appraisal is supporting the application of learning in practice. It is an opportunity for organisations to begin to measure the impact of their investment in education and training on organisational performance.

Anonymised data collected through the appraisal process can influence the commissioning of education and training, competence levels of managers, skill-mix of the workforce, change management programmes and corporate planning: financial, workforce and service delivery.

The appraisal process is so fundamental to an organisation's ability to achieve its objectives that it is strange that many view it as something they would invest more in if they had more time or fewer priorities. While organisations view the process in such limited ways appraisal will not give the return that it could to the organisation or individuals. Effective appraisals should be something that every organisation strives to deliver because of the return they give. Good practice in this area should be sought out and cascaded throughout the organisation. Effective appraisal may determine whether an organisation achieves its performance targets. Appraisal should be taken seriously and appropriate time and resources should be invested into doing it well.

Quality assurance

Appraisal processes need to be quality assured for the PCO to be able to demonstrate that it is protecting the public from poor or underperforming staff. Such quality assurance will relate to the appraisers, their training and support, as well as to systems to examine the quality of evidence in the documentation relating to staff performance and outcomes of personal development planning (PDP).

The NHS is becoming more aware of the need for quality assurance of educational provision, both of individual courses and by developing systems to accredit educational providers. In England, some of the Teaching PCTs, such as that in Stoke-on-Trent, are addressing this area, considering how to set up systems that consider the 'quality' of the trainers or tutors involved in design or delivery of a course, the extent to which the learning objectives and learning outcomes of a programme match the PDPs of individuals participating, and the strategies of PCOs or practices that are sponsoring the education. Such quality assurance should be integral to a clinical governance culture and the evaluation approach used, for example in evaluating the outcomes of PDPs (*see* Chapter 8 for more in-depth information on this).

Appraisal is an integral part of the clinical governance systems and culture in a PCO. The key principles of clinical governance are:

* a coherent approach to quality improvement
* clear lines of accountability for clinical quality systems
* effective processes for identifying and managing risk and addressing poor performance.

Context of appraisal and revalidation for doctors

The aims of the appraisal system are to give doctors an opportunity to discuss and receive regular feedback on their previous and continuing performance, and identify education and development needs, in whichever country in the UK they work.

The appraisal paperwork for doctors working in England, Scotland, Wales and Northern Ireland has been individualised by each country. The English version for GPs, for example, includes two extra sections to those of hospital consultants, management and research. The Scottish version focuses on core categories in preparation for revalidation of prescribing, referrals and peer review, clinical audit, significant event analysis and communication skills, summary of any complaints and other feedback.

In England, the responsibility for implementing GP appraisal has been placed with the PCTs. A national one-day training programme for appraisers was originally commissioned by the Department of Health for approximately three GP appraisers per PCT. This has since been supplemented by training provided through the Deaneries. It was intended that all GP principals would have been appraised by April 2003, but progress on implementing appraisal has been patchy and slow.

In Scotland, NHS Education for Scotland (NES) has overall national responsibility for GP appraisal. Appraisal will be the cornerstone for CPD for GPs in the future. Although the Health Boards employ the appraisers, NES is responsible for future design of the scheme and for the training of all appraisers. A practical handbook for appraisers and individuals being appraised has been produced, including standard feedback questionnaires for appraisers and those appraised as part of a quality assurance system for the scheme.[14]

In Wales, the National Assembly has agreed a service-level agreement with the Deanery to roll out the GP appraisal programme in 2003/04 based on the Wales pilot scheme.[15] The appraisers are selected, appointed, trained and paid by the Deanery, and the Deanery has produced a handbook.[16]

In Northern Ireland, appraisal will be the responsibility of the Local Health and Social Care Groups, once GPs join them. At present the project rests with the Health Boards. The Deanery is training appraisers, and hopes to provide quality assurance of the process and a support network for appraisers.

Appraisal and revalidation are based on the same sources of information – presented in the same structure as the seven main headings set out in the General Medical Council (GMC) guidance in *Good Medical Practice*.[17] The two processes perform different functions; appraisal is different from, but linked to, revalidation. Whereas revalidation involves an assessment against a standard of fitness to practise medicine, appraisal is concerned with the doctor's professional development within his or her working environment and the needs of the organisation for which the doctor works. *See* Table 1.1 for a comparison of appraisal and revalidation.[18]

Table 1.1:   Differences between appraisal and revalidation (SCHARR, 2001)[18]

Appraisal	*Revalidation*
• Employer led	• Profession led
• Local	• National
• Internal	• External
• Formative	• Summative
• Action oriented	• Status oriented
• Two-way process	• One-way process
• Annual	• Quinquennial

Whereas appraisal is a two-way process, with revalidation doctors will be regularly *required* to demonstrate that they are fit to practise. It seeks to identify poor perform-ance, makes judgements about doctors' fitness to practise and is a non-developmental process. Appraisal feeds into this by contributing to the information a doctor supplies for the revalidation process. Appraisal will provide a regular, structured recording system for documenting progress towards revalidation and identifying needs as part of the doctor's PDPs.

Appraisal and revalidation processes are being increasingly integrated. The PDP is a central part of the appraisal documentation, which will in turn be included in the portfolio of information available for revalidation. The revalidation portfolio will have supporting documents that include a record of developmental appraisals, clinical governance activities, outcomes of doctors' self-assessment of their performance and other work-based assessment, and evidence of CPD.[19]

Appraisal and professional regulation for healthcare professions

An overarching body, the Council for the Regulation of Healthcare Professions, was established in April 2003.[20] Its aim is to work with the existing regulatory bodies to build and manage a new framework for self-regulation that explicitly puts patients' interests first. The Council will enable co-ordination between the regulatory bodies and help to share good practice and information. The Council is independent from the government and directly answerable to Parliament. While it does not aim to get involved with the direct regulation of health professionals, it will have the power to refer unduly lenient decisions about professionals' fitness to practise to the High Court.

Co-regulation should become the guiding force of professional regulation in future. A standard of good practice that covers all health professionals should be developed. This is something the Council for the Regulation of Healthcare Professionals could be responsible for drawing up in future. It is envisaged that the Council will manage a framework of self-regulation that can accommodate new and emerging clinical roles that work across traditional professional divides, including the boundaries between health and social care.

Education, training and appraisal indicators in the new general medical services contract

The quality and outcomes framework of the new general medical services (GMS) contract includes 29 points across nine indicators. So, practice teams will be able to earn money from introducing a systematic approach to annual appraisals for all clinical and non-clinical team members. Box 1.4 describes the indicators and points available.

Box 1.4: Education, training and appraisal indicators for the GMS contract for general practice[21]

Indicators	*Points*
1 All practice-employed clinical staff have attended training/ updating in basic life support skills in previous 18 months	4
2 Practice undertaken minimum of six significant event reviews (SERs) in previous three years	4
3 All practice-employed nurses have an annual appraisal	2
4 All new staff receive induction training	3
5 All practice-employed staff attended training/updating in basic life support skills in previous three years	3
6 Practice does annual review of patient complaints and suggestions, and shares learning from them as a team	3
7 Practice has undertaken a minimum of 12 SERs in previous three years, including specified subjects	4
8 All practice-employed nurses have personal learning plans, reviewed at annual appraisal	3
9 All practice-employed non-clinical staff have annual appraisal	3

References

1 Department of Health (2002) *NHS Appraisal. Appraisal for general practitioners working in the NHS.* Department of Health, London. www.dh.gov.uk/PolicyAndGuidance/Human ResourcesAndTraining/LearningAndPersonalDevelopment/Appraisals/fs/en

2 Department of Health (1998) *A First Class Service.* Department of Health, London.

3 Nursing and Midwifery Council (2001) *The PREP Handbook.* Nursing and Midwifery Council, London.

4 Department of Health (1999) *Supporting Doctors, Protecting Patients.* Department of Health, London.

5 Jolly B and Grant J (1997) *The Good Assessment Guide.* Joint Centre for Education in Medicine, London.

6 Rowntree D (1982) *Evaluation and Improvement.* PCP Educational Series, London.

7 Miller GE (1990) The assessment of clinical skills/competence/performance. *Acad Med.* **65**: 563–7.

8 Wass V, Van der Vleuten CPM, Shatzer J and Jones R (2001) Assessment of clinical competence. *Lancet.* **357**: 945–9.

9 Stuart C (2003) *Assessment, Supervision and Support in Clinical Practice.* Churchill Livingstone, London.

10 Kirkpatrick DL (1967) *Evaluation of Training and Development Handbook.* McGraw-Hill, New York.

11 North Stoke Primary Care Trust (2003) *Appraisal Policy.* North Stoke PCT, Stoke-on-Trent.

12 Committee of General Practice Education Directors (COGPED) (2003) *Continuing Professional Development for General Practitioners.* A COGPED Position Paper. COGPED, London.

13 Improving Working Lives, www.dh.gov.uk/PolicyAndGuidance/HumanResourcesAndTraining/ModelEmployer/ImprovingWorkingLives/fs/en

14 NHS Education for Scotland (2003) *Appraisal for General Practitioners Working in Scotland.* NHS Scotland, Edinburgh.

15 Lewis M, Elwyn G and Wood F (2003) Appraisal of family doctors: an evaluation study. *BJGP.* **53**: 454–60.

16 Department of Postgraduate Education for General Practice (2003) *GP Appraisal in Wales.* Department of Postgraduate Education for General Practice, University of Wales College of Medicine, Cardiff.

17 General Medical Council (2002) *Good Medical Practice.* General Medical Council, London.

18 Martin D, Harrison P and Joesbury H (2003) *Extending Appraisal to all GPs.* ScHARR, University of Sheffield, Sheffield.

19 General Medical Council (2003) *A Licence to Practise & Revalidation.* General Medical Council, London.

20 Health Professions Council, www.hpc-uk.org/

21 General Practitioners Committee (GPC)/NHS Confederation (2003) *The New GMS Contract. Investing in General Practice.* GPC, London.

2

Making the most of your appraisal: when being appraised

To make the most of the opportunities for development that your appraisal should provide, you need to understand:

- the link between your continuing professional development (CPD) activities, personal development plan (PDP) and appraisal
- how to compile a portfolio that includes evidence of your learning and performance at work to discuss at your appraisal
- how to demonstrate your standards of practice
- tools and techniques to gather evidence of your performance at work for your appraisal portfolio
- what professional development activities can help you to be a more effective learner or professional when putting your appraisal action plan into practice
- how to prepare for your appraisal.

If both appraiser and individuals being appraised prepare well for the appraisal session, there will be no surprises – which might adversely affect the quality of the appraisal discussion.

You need to understand the difference between an appraisal and other types of review. The distinguishing characteristics have been picked out in Box 2.1.

Box 2.1: Distinguishing different aspects of performance review[1]

Appraisal (centred on person being appraised)
Involves reflection:

- Formative
- Developmental
- Confidential

Assessment (personal)
Involves measurement:

- Targets/audits/standards
- Complaints
- Significant events

continued overleaf

> **Performance management** (organisation)
> Involves comparison with others:
>
> • Assessment against organisational agenda
>
> **Revalidation** (external/public)
> Involves licensing:
>
> • Summative
> • Declaration of fitness to practise
> • Public

Linking your personal development plan to appraisal[2]

Learning involves many steps. It includes the acquisition of information, its retention, the ability to retrieve the information when needed and how to use that information for best practice. Demonstrating your learning involves being able to show the steps you have taken. Learning should be lifelong and encompass CPD.

CPD takes time, so it makes sense to optimise the time spent on CPD by overlapping learning undertaken to meet your personal and professional needs with that required for the performance of your role in the health service.

Many of those working in the health service have drawn up a PDP that is agreed with their line manager or local CPD tutor. Some have constructed their PDP in a systematic way and identified the priorities within it, or gathered evidence to demonstrate that what they have learnt was subsequently applied in practice. There is no uniform approach to the style or content of a PDP across different staff groups or health service settings. For some, a plan being drawn up is enough, while others encourage a systematic approach to identifying and addressing the individual's learning and service needs in order of importance or urgency.[3]

The new emphasis on accountability to the public in the NHS has given the PDP a higher profile and shown that it may be used in other ways. Many educationalists view a PDP as a tool to encourage individual staff to plan their own learning activities. The management view may be of a tool for quality assurance of staff performance. Health professionals may use their PDPs to strive to improve the quality of the care they deliver to patients and as a route to postgraduate awards or other health service-related quality awards.

The process of lifelong learning

For most health professional groups, CPD activities have traditionally been recorded as the number of hours undertaken rather than the gain in knowledge or skills achieved. For instance, the professional regulatory body for nursing, the Nursing and Midwifery Council (NMC), has stated within its Professional Code of Conduct (2002) that all registered nurses must maintain their professional knowledge and competence. The Code states that 'you should take part regularly in learning activities that develop your competence and performance'. This means that learning should be lifelong and encompass CPD.[4]

The formal requirements for nurses to reregister state that nurses must meet the post-registration education and practice standards (PREP). This includes completion of 750 hours in practice during the five years prior to renewal of registration, together with evidence that the nurse has met the professional standards for CPD. This standard comprises a minimum of five days' (or 35 hours') learning activity relevant to the nurse's clinical practice in the three years prior to the renewal of his or her professional registration. Many nurses see this requirement as inadequate, as they undertake much more CPD than this to keep themselves abreast of current changes in practice.[5]

However, some nurses pay little attention to the recording of their CPD activity. Until recently, most nurses did not reflect on what they learnt or whether they applied it in practice. They did not see the necessity for protected time for learning and reflection among their everyday responsibilities, or target their time and effort on priority topics. Times are changing, and with the introduction of PDPs and appraisals or individual performance reviews, nurses are realising that they must take a more professional approach to learning and document their standards of competence, performance and service delivery.

Your personal development plan

Your personal development plan will be an integral part of your future appraisal portfolio to demonstrate your fitness to practise as a health professional or your performance at work.

Your initial plan should:

*   identify your gaps or weaknesses in knowledge, skills or attitudes
*   specify topics for learning as a result of changes: in your role, responsibilities, the organisation in which you work
*   link into the learning needs of others in your workplace or team of colleagues
*   tie in with the service development priorities of your practice, the primary care organisation (PCO) or the NHS as a whole
*   describe how you identified your learning needs
*   set your learning needs and associated goals in order of importance and urgency
*   justify your selection of learning goals
*   describe how you will achieve your goals and over what time period
*   describe how you will evaluate the learning outcomes you set in your PDP.

Each year you will continue or revise your PDP. It should demonstrate how you carried out your learning and evaluation plans, show that you have learnt what you set out to do (or why it was modified) and how you applied your new learning in practice. In addition, you will find that you have new priorities and fresh learning needs as circumstances change.

***

Box 2.2: Tips on maintaining a worthwhile PDP – a senior manager's perspective[6]

1   Learn a new competence every six months
2   Transfer an existing competence to a new circumstance or setting
3   Extend your network of people to help your development
4   Write something to change people's minds
5   Publish something, e.g. a letter, to share knowledge or influence others
6   Look after your work/life balance

The main task is to capture what you have learned, in a way that suits you, just as the manager whose tips are listed in Box 2.2 does. Then you can look back at what you have done and:

- reflect on it later and decide to learn more or make changes as a result, and identify further needs
- demonstrate to others that you are fit to practise or work through:
  - what you have done
  - what you have learnt
  - what changes you have made as a result
  - the standards of work you have achieved and are maintaining
  - how you monitor your performance at work
- use it to show how your personal learning fits in with the requirements of your practice or the NHS, and other people's personal and professional development plans.

Prepare your portfolio

Use your portfolio of evidence of what you have learnt and your standards of practice to:

- identify significant experiences to serve as important sources of learning
- reflect on the learning that arose from those experiences
- demonstrate learning in practice
- analyse and identify further learning needs and ways in which these needs can be met.

Organise all the evidence of your learning into a CPD portfolio of some sort. It is up to you how you keep this record of your learning. Examples include the following.

- *An ongoing learning journal* in which you draw up and describe your plan, record how you determined your needs and prioritised them, report why you attended particular educational meetings or courses and what you got out of them, as well as the continuing cycle of review, making changes and evaluating them.
- *An A4 file* with lots of plastic sleeves into which you build up a systematic record of your educational activities in line with your plan.
- *A box*: chuck in everything to do with your learning plan as you do it and sort it out into a sensible order every few months with a good review once a year.

Your documentation might include all sorts of things, not just formal audits – although they make a good start. It might include reports of educational activities attended, statements of your roles and responsibilities, copies of publications you have read and critically appraised, and reports of your work. You could incorporate observations by others, evaluations of you observing other colleagues and how their practice differs from yours, descriptions of self-improvements, a video of a typical activity, materials that demonstrate your skills to others, products of your input or learning – a new protocol for example. Box 2.3 gives a list of material you might include in your portfolio.

Box 2.3:   Possible contents of a portfolio

- Workload logs
- Case descriptions
- Videos
- Audiotapes
- Patient satisfaction surveys
- Research surveys
- Report of change or innovation
- Commentaries on published literature or books
- Records of critical incidents and learning points
- Notes from formal teaching sessions with reference to clinical work or other evidence

---

When you are preparing to submit the portfolio for a discussion with a colleague (e.g. at an appraisal) or assessment (e.g. for a university postgraduate award or revalidation), write a self-assessment of your previous action plan. You might integrate your self-assessment into your PDP to show what you have achieved and what gaps you have still to address. Decide where you are now and where you want to be in one, three or five years' time. Select items from your portfolio for inclusion for each part of the documentation – you might have one compartment of your portfolio per specialty topic, or if you are a doctor, you might organise section headings according to those in *Good Medical Practice*[7] (*see* page 18).

Index your learning steps and your standards of practice and cross-reference them to the relevant sections of the paperwork. Discuss the contents of your portfolio with a colleague or a mentor to gain other people's perspectives of your work and look for blind spots.

Include evidence of your competence as a practitioner with a special interest[2,8]

You may have a particular expertise or special interest in a clinical field or non-clinical area such as management, teaching or research. It may be that you have a lead role or responsibility in your practice for chronic disease management of clinical conditions such as diabetes, asthma, mental health or coronary heart disease. Or you may be employed by a PCO or hospital trust as a practitioner with a special interest (PwSI) to:

- lead in the development of services
- deliver a procedure-based service
- deliver an opinion-based service.

There is little consistency in extent of training or qualifications at present within or across the various PwSI specialty areas.[8,9] Whatever your role or responsibility or expertise, your portfolio should include examples of evidence that show that you are competent, and that you have a consistently good performance in your specialty area. You may have parallel appraisals that you can include from another employer – for example, the university if you have a research or teaching post, or a hospital consultant if he or she supervises you in a clinical specialty.

Link evidence of your professional developments to the new general medical services (GMS) contract or personal medical services (PMS) practice arrangements

The areas within the quality framework on the new GMS contract will probably be the ones that you prioritise in your PDP when looking at your service development needs.[10] The four main components of the quality framework are all relevant to your personal and professional development.

The NMC sets out standards that must be met as part of the duties and responsibilities of nurses in the Professional Code of Conduct.[4] The clauses within the Code have been drawn up to create expectations for the public relating to the behaviour they can expect from nurses, and to create a uniform standard of behaviour with which all nurses must comply. A good portfolio should reflect these standards of care wherever possible; for example, confidential information should be protected. Therefore, if your portfolio includes reflective writing there should be no way of identifying specific patients. The clauses within the Code of Conduct are shared values from all the UK healthcare regulatory bodies.

Doctors must be able to meet these standards with a record of their own performance in their revalidation portfolio if they want to retain a licence to practise. The nine key headings of expected standards of practice for all GPs working in England that any other health professional might also address are as follows.

1 *Good professional practice.* This relates to clinical care, keeping records (including writing reports and keeping colleagues informed), access and availability, treatment in emergencies and making effective use of resources.
2 *Maintaining good medical practice.* This includes keeping up to date and maintaining your performance.
3 *Relationships with patients.* This encompasses providing information about your services, maintaining trust, avoiding discrimination and prejudice against patients, relating well to patients and apologising if things go wrong.
4 *Working with colleagues.* This relates to working with colleagues, working in teams, referring patients and accepting posts.
5 *Teaching and training, appraising and assessing.* You may be in a position to teach or train colleagues or students, and appraise or assess peers, employees or students.
6 *Probity* includes providing true information about your services, honesty in financial and commercial dealings, and providing references.
7 *Health* can include how you overcome or compensate your own health problems, or help with or address health problems in other doctors.
8 *Research.* Conducting research in an ethical manner.
9 *Management.* The section on management concerns any responsibility GPs have for management outside the practice. GPs might wish to include management responsibilities that cross the interface between their practice and PCO.

Professional competence is the first area of concern to employers and the public. You should be able to demonstrate that you can maintain a satisfactory standard of clinical care most of the time in your everyday work. Some of the time you will be brilliant, of course! Celebrate those moments. On other occasions, you or others around you will be critical of your performance and feel that you could have done much better. Reflect on those episodes to learn from them.

Ten examples of tools and techniques to provide evidence of your performance at work for your appraisal portfolio[3]

When you gather evidence of your performance at work, try to document as many aspects of your work at one time as you can, so that for example an audit covers as many of the key headings from *Good Medical Practice*[7] as possible. When you are identifying what you need to learn, or gaps in service delivery, make sure that you involve patients and show how you interact with the team. This gives you evidence about 'relationships with patients' and 'working with colleagues', as well as the clinical area that you are focusing on or auditing.

Determine what it is that you 'don't know you don't know' by:

• asking patients, users and non-users of your service
• comparing your performance with best practice or that of peers
• comparing your performance with objectives in business plans or national directives
• asking colleagues from different disciplines about shortfalls in how your work interfaces with theirs.

1 Compare your performance against protocols or guidelines

Are you familiar with all the protocols or guidelines that are used by someone, somewhere in the primary care team? You might determine your learning needs and those of other primary care team members by piling all the protocols or guidelines that exist in your practice in a big heap and rationalising them so that you have a common set across the practice. Working as a team you can compare your own knowledge and usual practice with others, and with protocols or guidelines recommended by the National Institute for Clinical Excellence (NICE)[11] or National Service Frameworks or the Scottish Intercollegiate Guideline Network (SIGN).[12]

Alternatively, you might compare your own practice with a protocol or guideline that is generally accepted at a national or local level. You could audit the standard of your practice to find out how often you adhere to such a protocol or guideline, and if you can justify why you deviate from the recommendations.

2 Undertake audit

Audit is:

> the method used by health professionals to assess, evaluate, and improve the care of patients in a systematic way, to enhance their health and quality of life.[13]

The five stages in the audit cycle are to:

1 describe the criteria and standards you are trying to achieve
2 measure your current performance of how well you are providing care or services in an objective way
3 compare your performance with criteria and standards

4   identify the need for change – to performance, adjustment of criteria or standards, resources, available data
5   make any required changes as necessary and re-audit later.

For the purposes of audit, performance or practice is often broken down into the three aspects of structure, process and outcome. Structural audits might concern considering resources such as equipment, premises, skills, people, etc. Process audits focus on what is done to the patient, e.g. clinical protocols and guidelines. Audits of outcomes consider the impact of care or services on the patient, and might include patient satisfaction, health gains and effectiveness of care or services. You might look at aspects of quality of the structure, process and outcome of the delivery of any clinical field, focusing on access, equity of care between different groups in the population, efficiency, economy, effectiveness for individual patients, etc.[13]

Set standards for your performance, find out how you are doing, search to find out best practice, make the changes and then re-audit the care given to patients in the future with the same problem. Some variations on audit include the following.

- *Case note analysis.* This gives an insight into your current practice. It might be a retrospective review of a random selection of notes or a prospective survey of consecutive patients with the same condition as they present to see you.
- *Peer review.* Compare an area of practice with other individual professionals or managers; or compare practice teams as a whole. An independent body might compare all practices in one area, e.g. within a PCT or PCO, so that like is compared with like.
- *Criteria-based audit.* This compares clinical practice with specific standards, guidelines or protocols. Re-audit of changes should demonstrate improvements in the quality of patient care.
- *External audit.* Prescribing advisors or managers in PCOs can supply information about indicators of performance for audit. Visits from external bodies such as the Healthcare Commission expose the PCO or hospital trust in England and Wales to external audit.
- *Significant event audit.* Think of an incident where a patient or you experienced an adverse event. This might be an unexpected death, an unplanned pregnancy, an avoidable side effect from prescribed medication, a violent attack on a member of staff, or an angry outburst in public by you or a work colleague. You can review the case and reflect on the sequence of events that led to that critical event occurring. It is likely that there were a multitude of factors leading up to that significant event. You should take the case to a multidisciplinary meeting to reflect and analyse what were the triggers, causes and consequences of the event. Complete the significant event audit cycle by planning what individuals or the practice as a whole might do to avoid a similar event happening in future. This might include undertaking further learning and/or making appropriate changes to the practice or your systems.
  - Step 1: describe who was involved, the time of day, the task/activity, the context and any other relevant information.
  - Step 2: discuss the reasons for the event or situation arising with other colleagues, review case notes or other records.
  - Step 3: reflect on the effects of the event on the participants and the professionals involved.
  - Step 4: decide how you or others might have behaved differently. Describe your options for how the procedures at work might be changed to minimise or eliminate the event from recurring.

- Step 5: plan changes that are needed, how they will be implemented, who will be responsible for what and when, what further training or resources are required. Then carry out the changes.
- Step 6: re-audit later to see whether changes to procedures or new knowledge and skills are having the desired effects. Give feedback to the primary care team.

3 Assessment by an external body

A traditional way of showing that you are competent is by taking and passing an examination. It is a good way of testing recalled knowledge in a written or oral examination, or establishing how you behave in a clinical situation on the day of a practical examination, but may not relate to real life. A summative examination (i.e. done at the end of a course of study) gives a measure of your learning up to that date.

You might undertake an objective test of your knowledge and skills. Examples are a computer-based test in the form of multiple choice questions and patient management problems. The Royal College of General Practitioners' (RCGP) series of quality awards provide external assessment – Membership by Assessment of Performance, Fellowship by Assessment, Quality Team Development, etc. Trained assessors will give feedback to individual doctors or practice teams about their performance compared with set standards and their peers.

4 Eliciting the views of patients

You might assess patients' satisfaction with:

- you
- your practice
- the local hospital's way of working
- other services available in your locality.

Avoid surveys where questions are relatively superficial or biased. A more specific enquiry should uncover particular elements of patients' dissatisfaction, which will be more useful if you are trying to identify your learning needs. Use a well-validated patient questionnaire instead of risking producing your own ambiguous or flawed version, such as the General Practice Assessment Questionnaire (GPAQ – *see* www. npcrdc.man.ac.uk) or the Doctors' Interpersonal Skills Questionnaire (DISQ – *see* website www.ex.ac.uk/cfep). Many doctors and practice teams have already used these patient survey methods, providing a bank of data against which to compare your performance.

Other sources of feedback from patients might be obtained through suggestion boxes for patients to contribute comments, or the practice team recording all patients' suggestions and complaints, however trivial, looking for patterns in the comments received.

There will be learning to be had from every complaint – even if the complaint does not have any substance, there should be something to learn about the shortfall in communication between you and the complainant.

The evolving of the 'expert patient programme' should mean that there is a pool of well-informed patients with chronic conditions who can contribute their insights into what you (or the service) need to learn from a patient's perspective.[14]

5 Observing your work environment and role

Observation could be informal and opportunistic, or more systematic working through a structured checklist. One method of self-assessment might be to audiotape yourself at work dealing with patients (after obtaining patients' informed consent). Listen to the tape afterwards to review your communication and consultation skills – on your own or with a friend or colleague. If you have access to video equipment, you might use that instead.

Look at the equipment in your practice. Do you know how to operate it properly? Assess yourself undertaking practical procedures or ask someone to watch you operate the equipment or undertaking the practical procedure and give you feedback about your performance.

6 Reading and reflecting

When reading articles in respected journals reflect on what the key messages mean for you in your situation. Note down topics about which you know little but are relevant to your work, and calculate if you have further learning needs not met by the article you are reading. If the article is relevant to your practice, record what changes you will make and how you will make the changes. Record how you share your newly gained knowledge with others in your practice or team.

7 Monitor access and availability to healthcare

Access and availability

You could look at waiting times to see a health professional. Compare results at intervals (a spreadsheet is a good way to do this). Do you or other staff have learning needs in relation to the use of technology, or new ways of redesigning the service you offer?

Referrals to other agencies and hospitals

You might audit and re-audit the time taken from the date the patient is seen to:

- the referral being sent (do you need more secretarial time?)
- the date the patient is seen by the other agency (could the patient be seen elsewhere quicker or do you need to liaise with other agencies over referrals?)
- the date the patient's needs have been met by investigation, diagnosis, treatment, provision of aid or support, etc. (can you influence how quickly these are completed?).

Identify any learning needs here. For instance, new methods of teamwork with a different mix of skills between doctors, nurses and non-clinically qualified assistants could provide extra services in the practice, or you might retrain to become a practitioner with a special clinical interest.

8 Assess risk[15]

There are five steps to risk assessment:

1 Look for and list the hazards.

2   Decide who might be harmed and how.
3   Evaluate the risks arising from the hazards and decide whether existing precautions are adequate or more should be done.
4   Record the findings.
5   Review the findings of your risk assessment from time to time and revise it if necessary.

You do not want to spend a lot of time and effort identifying risks or making changes if they do not matter much. When you have identified a risk, consider:

* is the risk large?
* does it happen often?
* is it a significant risk?

Risks may be prevented, avoided, minimised or managed where they cannot be eliminated. You may need to learn how to do this.

9 Consider your patient population's health needs

Create a detailed profile of your patient population. Ask your PCO or public health lead for information about your patient population and/or comparative information about the general population living in the district – morbidity and mortality statistics, referral patterns, age/sex-mix, ethnicity and population trends.

Include information about the wider determinants of health, such as housing, numbers of the population in, and types of, employment, geographical location, the environment, crime and safety, educational attainment and socio-economic data. Make a note of any particular health problems, such as higher-than-average teenage pregnancy rates or drug misuse. Focus on the current state of health inequalities within your patient population or between your patient population and the district as a whole.

10 Assess the quality of your services

Quality may be subdivided into eight components:

* equity
* access
* acceptability and responsiveness
* appropriateness
* communication
* continuity
* effectiveness
* efficiency.[16]

Look for service development needs reflecting why patients receive a poor quality of service, such as:

* inadequately trained staff or staff with poor levels of competence
* lack of confidentiality
* staff not being trained in the management of emergency situations
* doctors or nurses not being contactable, or being ineffective, in an emergency

- treatment being unavailable due to poor management of resources or services
- insufficient numbers of available staff for the workload
- arrangements for transfer of information from one team member to another being inadequate
- team members not acting on information received.

Professional development activities to help you be a more effective learner or professional

Learning styles

Everyone has his or her preferred learning style(s). You will be likely to learn more effectively if you find ways that suit you, and teachers that match your own preferred learning style(s). Honey and Mumford have described four learning styles:[17]

Activists like to be fully involved in new experiences, open-minded, will try anything once, thrive on the challenge of new experiences but soon get bored and want to go on to the next challenge. They are gregarious and like to be the centre of attention. Activists learn best through new experiences, short activities, situations where they can be centre stage (chairing meetings, leading discussions), when allowed to generate new ideas and have a go at things or brainstorm ideas.

Reflectors like to stand back, think about things thoroughly and collect a lot of information before coming to a conclusion. They are cautious, take a back seat in meetings and discussions, adopt a low profile, and appear tolerant and unruffled. When they do act it is by using the wide picture of their own and others' views. Reflectors learn best from situations where they are allowed to watch and think about activities before acting. They carry out research first of all, review evidence, produce carefully constructed reports and can reach decisions in their own time.

Theorists like to adapt and integrate observations into logical maps and models, using step-by-step processes. They tend to be perfectionists, and are detached, analytical and objective. They reject anything that is subjective, flippant and lateral thinking in nature. Theorists learn best from activities where there are plans, maps and models to describe what is going on. When they are offered complex situations to understand they prefer to take time to explore the methodology, work with structured situations with a clear purpose and be intellectually stretched.

Pragmatists like to try out ideas, theories and techniques to see if they work in practice. They will act quickly and confidently on ideas that attract them and are impatient with ruminating and open-ended discussions. They are down-to-earth people who like solving problems and making practical decisions, responding to problems as a challenge. Pragmatists learn best when there is an obvious link between the subject and their jobs. They enjoy trying out techniques with coaching and feedback, practical issues, real problems to solve and when they are given the immediate chance to implement what has been learned.

Activity 2.1

To self-assess your learning style you should complete the 80-item Learning Styles questionnaire[17] or attend a course that includes rating your learning style as an integral part.

Time management[18]

Better time management is often a skill that those being appraised prioritise in their PDP. The many ways to manage your time better fall into three main categories.

- *Reducing the amount of work to be done* by refusing it in the first place, delegating it, or doing less of it.
- *Doing the work more quickly* by doing it less thoroughly or processing it more efficiently.
- *Allowing more time for a particular piece of work* so that there is less time pressure on completing it.

Prioritise your time. Do not allow yourself or others to waste it. The first step is to be clear about your goals in your work and home lives, or leisure. Then you need to structure sufficient time around those priorities. If you have a choice about whether or not to carry out an activity, match it against your goals. If doing it takes you further away from your goals then refuse to take it on, but if it coincides with your goals, consider if you have time to fit it in.

Make sure you spend your quality time doing the most important or complex jobs. It is too easy to focus on getting small, unimportant tasks done and put off tackling the big ones, which just hang over you and make you feel guilty for leaving them unattended. A high-priority task has to be done, a medium-priority job may be delegated and a low-priority task should only be done if you have no medium- or high-priority tasks waiting, or you are too jaded to tackle them. The majority of your time should be devoted to pursuing your most important goals, and a small proportion of your time spent on less-important matters.

Control interruptions. Interruptions are one of the biggest timewasters, especially if someone else could have handled the problem or taken the message, or no action was required. Even if an interruption is necessary it may occur at the wrong time, wrecking your concentration or train of thought. Agree rules in your workplace for who may be interrupted and when. You will achieve more in designated sessions of quiet, uninterrupted periods than in a longer allotment of time broken up by various activities. You need uninterrupted time for concentrating on planning, writing reports or analysing progress.

Include sufficient time for thinking, doing, meeting, developing and learning. You need to be fresh and creative to stay on top of the demands made on you. You can only manage this in the longer term if you have the right mix of stimulating work, personal and professional development, and networking regularly timetabled into your daily schedule.

Try to allow at least 10% of your time for dealing with unexpected tasks. In the unlikely event that everything goes smoothly and you do not need the extra time, it will be a bonus to have that additional space to catch up on the backlog of paperwork.

Delegate whatever and however you can. Only accept delegated work if you have the necessary skills, time and experience. If you are in a position to delegate work and responsibilities, decide what only *you* can do and delegate as much of the rest as possible to others. If you are more usually on the receiving end of delegated work, try to make sure you understand what is required, and that you have the necessary time, skills and experience, before agreeing or acquiescing to take on the new work. If you don't have the relevant time or skills, negotiate in your most assertive manner how you will get the training and when you will do the work.

Do not just consider delegation at work, but at home too – cleaning, gardening, help from all the family, etc.

Control your work flow. Concentrate on one task at a time. Complete it and either move on to another job or take a short break to refresh yourself and clear your mind ready to start again. Do not switch between tasks as you will waste effort having to start thinking about the topic all over again each time you take it up.

You are likely to be more efficient if you group small similar tasks together, such as returning phonecalls. Always have one or two small jobs put by or carried with you, so that if you are kept waiting you can get on with those jobs and not waste time. Maintain control of your paperwork. Do not let it build up so that you feel overwhelmed, or you will put off tackling it at all or work more slowly as the enormity of the task depresses you.

Minimise paperwork. Only pick up each piece of paper once, and only start a job when you have time to finish it. Deal with the most complicated task first, while you are fresh, and delegate appropriately as far as possible.

Sort paperwork into:

- must be done today
- can wait a few days
- can wait a few weeks
- for someone else to do.

Activity 2.2: Keep a log of daily activities

Photocopy the daily log overleaf. Record all your activities each day for a week, including an off-duty period if possible. Then sort the activities into three separate columns:

- *personal needs*, including shopping, sleeping, domestic chores, bodily needs, etc.
- *work*, including reading work-related books, reports and papers
- *leisure*, including sport, relaxation, reading, music, etc.

Once you have worked out totals for the types of activity for each day, group the activities within the categories personal needs, work and leisure. Compare several days of daily recordings for these categories with the Health Education Authority's (now the Health Development Agency) recommendations for a healthy lifestyle:[18]

- 45–55% on personal needs
- 25–30% on work
- 20–25% on leisure.

Look for any trends or patterns of activities in the daily time logs – such as staying late at work or catching up on paperwork at home. Do you think you can improve the way you divide your own time? Could you change the balance in the way you allocate time to essential, desirable and unimportant activities? Discuss your log with your partner or family at home, or a work colleague.

Daily log of activities

Time spent (to nearest quarter of an hour) on					
Personal needs (shopping, washing, domestic chores, sleeping)		Work		Leisure	
Activity	Time spent	Activity	Time spent	Activity	Time spent
Total/day		Total/day		Total/day	

Activity 2.3: Reduce time pressures at work

Use this activity to look at the suggestions for reducing the time pressures listed below from the perspectives of an individual and an organisation.

What you can do as an individual	*What the organisation can do*
Plan well in advance to avoid crises	Plan well in advance to avoid crises
Allow 10% of your time for unexpected tasks	Organise time management training for staff
Do not book a meeting too close to a previous commitment that may overrun	Match staff numbers to volume of work
Build in time for reflection and planning	Organise realistic work plans
Minimise interruptions	Discourage social chit-chat in work time
Make maximum use of technology	Make maximum use of technology
Other:	Other:

Action points to reduce time pressures
What you will do:

As an individual	*And when*	*As an organisation*	*And when*
1			
2			
3			
4			
5			

Undertaking this activity will force you to realise the varied solutions available for reducing time pressures and that you are not helpless. It will also help you to understand that you cannot reduce time pressures on you as an individual in isolation from the rest of the team or organisation. The individual and organisation need to work together to reduce time pressures effectively.

Keeping a reflective learning log[19]

Do not restrict yourself to a particular event. You can use the log to record your other thoughts, ideas, insights and feelings. You might also record what worked for you and what did not, and the reasons for that. Using a reflective log in this way will help you to become more aware of how and what you are learning.

Activity 2.4

You can use your reflective learning log to pick out the most personally significant experiences on a particular day and record what you learned from the experience(s). This will involve reflecting on:

- what was most significant
- why this was personally significant
- what you learned
- any actions you propose to take as a result.

Stress management[18]

The types of practical method you can use to cope with stress at work include:

- seeking support from colleagues
- sharing problems with colleagues
- adopting better time-management practices
- more appropriate booking times for appointments and meetings
- increasing the amount of protected time off-duty, limiting working hours to those for which you are contracted
- admitting and discussing doubts and worries with others
- achieving a better balance between work and home commitments.

It is not stress itself that is necessarily the damaging factor but your inability to cope with it. In a changing world people need to learn new ways of coping. Only you can identify the best stress managing solutions for you. Think of:

- preventive strategies, i.e. reduce or change the nature or frequency of the source(s) of stress
- altering your individual response to stress or improving the practice's ability to recognise and deal with stress-related problems as they arise
- minimising the effects of stress, i.e. working with colleagues as a team to relieve pressure through good communication, delegation, debriefing and support, etc.

Activity 2.5: Undertake your own significant event audit of stress from work

Analyse a significant event at work (*see* pages 20–1).

- Step 1: Write down a factual account of the stressful situation you have chosen – who was involved, the time of day and the task/activity you or others were doing.

- Step 2: Write down the reasons for the stressful situation arising.

- Step 3: Write down the effects of stress on you or others involved in the situation you have chosen.

- Step 4: Record how you or others might have behaved differently, or how the organisation might be changed to reduce or eliminate this cause of stress from recurring.

- Step 5: Analyse the significant event with a colleague to gain further insights and perspectives, plus new ideas for solutions and help with putting them into practice. Plan changes and put them into operation.

Be assertive[18]

Assertiveness is about knowing and practising your rights – to change your mind, to make mistakes, to refuse demands, to express emotions, to be yourself without having to act for other people's benefit, and to make decisions or statements without having always to justify them. It takes practice to be assertive – so get some practice in at work and at home. The biggest challenge may be being assertive with yourself so that you do not agree to take on additional tasks that are not essential for you to undertake, or that fall outside your own priority areas.

How often do you hear people saying: 'No, no ... no ... oh alright then, I suppose so'? Listen carefully to what is being asked of you, weigh up the time, effort and skills the task or activity will take, and the extent to which it is an essential, desirable or possible feature of your working or home lives – and then decide on your assertive response.

Twelve key points to remember about being assertive.

1   Say 'No' clearly and then move away or change the subject. Keep repeating 'No' – do not be diverted.
2   Be honest and direct with everyone.
3   Do not apologise or justify yourself more than is reasonable.
4   Offer a workable compromise and negotiate an agreement that suits you and the other party.
5   Pause before answering with a 'Yes' you will regret. Delay your response and give yourself more time to think by asking for more information.
6   Be aware of your body language and keep it as assertive as possible. Match your tone to your words (do not smile if you are giving a serious message).
7   Use the 'broken record' technique – repeat your same message persistently in a calm manner to someone who is trying to pressurise you. Do not be side-tracked.
8   Show that you are listening to the other person's point of view and giving them a fair hearing.
9   Practise expressing your opinion and rights rather than expecting other people to guess what you want.
10 Do not be too hard on yourself if you make a mistake – everyone is human.
11 Be confident enough to change your mind if that is appropriate.
12 Remember that it can be assertive to say nothing.

Activity 2.6

Consider whether your 'body language' reinforces your attempts to be assertive when in situations where you disagree with others over an issue that you consider to be important.

Non-verbal behaviour: the body language that gives you away

Passive	Assertive	Aggressive
Covers mouth with hand	Direct eye contact	Gesticulates expansively
Looks down at the floor	Head erect	Clenched/pounding fists
Constant shifting of weight	Descriptive hand gestures	Finger pointing

continued overleaf

Fiddles with clothing	Emphasises key words	Hands on hips
Rubs head or parts of body	Steady, firm voice	Rigid posture
Frequent nodding of head	Open movements	Strident voice
Throat clearing	Relaxed	Stares others down

Do you recognise your non-verbal behaviour patterns from the list above as mainly 'passive', 'assertive' or 'aggressive' in a:

*   situation at work with a patient?
*   situation at work with other colleagues?

Are you consistent? Do you behave differently at work from how you do at home or in another setting? Could you change your non-verbal behaviour and the signals you give out so that you behave more consistently?

Seek support[18]

Research into stress has shown that people with the best social support network who interact well with other people are able to cope with stress and are the least affected by it. Be prepared to ask for help. That is not a sign of weakness or ignorance. Support networks may be used for another professional opinion or for emotional assistance. Support for colleagues should be non-judgemental and a culture developed at work where people do not feel embarrassed or silly to be asking for help.

Activity 2.7

Draw up a personal map of support mechanisms in your life. Undertaking this exercise will help you to realise for yourself the components of your life that lend you support, and that you can build on.

*   Stage 1: Draw yourself in the middle of a piece of plain paper. Then draw pictures to represent all the sources of support in your life – people, things, situations, environment, etc. Link each picture to you in the centre with a line (*see* Figure 2.1 for example).
*   Stage 2: Next add in drawings of what other sources of support you have used in the past but not employed for a while, and add other pictures of what extra sources of support you would like to have. Link each picture to you in the centre of the page.
*   Stage 3: Draw in the barriers that stop you from using these sources of support, across the line linking that particular source with you.
*   Stage 4: Share and compare your personal support map with someone else. Discuss your various sources of support, which ones you would like to enhance, the presence of the barriers that stop you making more of your sources of support, what is missing and what action you can take to improve your situation. Make a plan to remove at least one barrier and enhance or create at least one source of support.

continued opposite

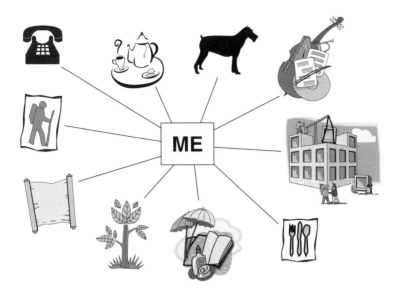

Figure 2.1:   Example of Stage 1 of a personal support map (contributed by Schwartz A[20]).

Now draw your own support map. Can you increase the number and types of support in your life?

Raise your self-esteem

Even confident seeming people may suffer from low self-esteem. Some people working in the NHS blame the hierarchical systems for contributing to their loss of self-esteem. You can deliberately raise your self-esteem by positive tactics and thinking. But, to effect any change you have to be prepared to take the risk of failure – success is not automatic. And to ride failures successfully you have to develop a positive approach before you start so that you can set yourself up to learn from failure rather than be cast down by it.

Ten positive strategies to raise your self-esteem.

1 Accept that not every attempt to change will be a success.
2 Be prepared to take a risk to effect a change in your life.
3 Try positive visualisation, that is imagine yourself successfully managing a forthcoming event or activity about which you are feeling apprehensive.
4 Use positive body language – people will treat you more positively too.
5 Review and recall past successes and hold them in the forefront of your mind.
6 Learn from any mistakes or failures.
7 Learn to feel comfortable with yourself – physically and mentally.
8 Write your worries down and review them periodically rather than continually fretting over them.
9 Be aware of your good points and constantly reinforce them in your thinking.
10 Do the best for yourself and give yourself every opportunity to succeed – do not set yourself up to fail.

Activity 2.8: Review the state of your self-esteem

Do you need to raise your self-esteem? If so, write down any positive strategies you could use to raise your self-esteem. If your self-esteem is reasonably good, what can you do to maintain it? What will you do and when?

1

2

3

4

Make a plan to review the outcomes of this exercise.

Preparing for your appraisal

Effective appraisal depends on both you and your appraiser preparing for the appraisal interview in advance. There should be an opportunity for you both to exchange information and documents before the interview. The appraiser should understand the pressures that the demands of patient care and limited resources create for you. He or she should be able to make allowances for any issues or problems that you have had in your everyday work that are beyond your control. You need to collect facts about any such pressures or resource problems, rather than impressions. Be specific rather than whinge. Then your evidence about the barriers that inhibit you and other colleagues from achieving best practice can be collated to inform business planning and the workforce and educational strategies of your PCO or PCT.

If you record your personal and professional development activities throughout the year under the same headings required for your appraisal documentation, you should avoid unnecessary work in preparing your appraisal portfolio and re-arranging the information and evidence that you have gathered for other purposes. So collate evidence of your performance and develop a personal portfolio that includes details of your personal development plan: identified needs, learning plan, changes made to service delivery as a result, etc., as the recommendation in Box 2.4 describes.

Box 2.4

'One thing we have learnt is that it is far better to collect your evidence for the appraisal process over the course of the year than to try to find it just before a session is booked ... Certainly where this has been done rigorously, it makes the appraisal process very efficient and straightforward.'[21]

It may take considerable time to complete your organisation's appraisal forms. Allow at least four hours, and even more time than this if you know that you are not good at completing forms, or if you have had little previous experience of preparing for such a review and assessment of your work. Use that time to reflect on what you have achieved in the past year or since you last updated your PDP.

Do not repeat the same information in different sections of the forms unnecessarily. Be as brief or as lengthy in your responses as is appropriate to the information that you have to convey – but try to keep to the point. Your appraiser will be looking for evidence of your assertions in the supporting documentation and through discussion with you. The reports or documents you assemble in support of your appraisal forms should be listed and cross-referenced.

Make the most of your appraisal discussion by putting your trust into the process and the appraiser, and make the system work for you. You should expect a fair hearing from your appraiser, who should have been trained to carry out appraisal. If you do not believe that appraisal will be a meaningful process in which you can trust the colleague who will be appraising your work, you may be driven to conceal particular areas where your work or performance is imperfect. If you prioritise areas to learn more about that build entirely on your strengths rather than addressing your weaknesses, your PDP will be meaningless.

What qualities should you expect in your appraiser?

The suggested lists of essential and desirable attributes given in Box 2.5 have been derived from a variety of sources. Some of these qualities will be more important than others to how well your appraisal goes and what benefits come out of it – for you and the NHS as a whole.

Box 2.5: Qualities of an effective appraiser

Essential
- Impartial
- Good listener
- Supportive
- Trustworthy
- Interested
- Perceptive
- Self-aware
- Respected
- Ethical
- Respectful
- An effective leader
- Skilled in feedback
- Chemistry: intellectual and emotional compatibility
- Able to challenge
- Non-judgemental
- Confidential
- Committed to their own personal and professional development
- Has time and energy to fulfil their contract with you
- Understands your work or discipline
- Understands how and where the organisation in which you work is going

Desirable
- Knowledge
- Technical expertise
- Experience
- Inspiring
- Patient
- Advisor
- Seniority
- Knows the health service
- Able to receive feedback

Countdown to your appraisal

The exchanging of information in the completed appraisal paperwork between you and your appraiser should take place in good time for your appraisal meeting – aim for three or so weeks before. You will send your appraiser your completed appraisal forms and supporting documentation, and your appraiser should let you have a copy of any information he or she has about your performance. This should give you time to collect additional evidence if you think the appraiser's information is incorrect or misleading. It gives you an opportunity to reflect on the likely content and outcomes of the forthcoming appraisal discussion. Similarly, the appraiser can familiarise him or herself with the information about your practice and can start thinking through the main issues, ready for the appraisal discussion.

Three weeks before at the latest:

- complete your appraisal forms (hopefully electronically) and send in to your appraiser (by email/post), retaining a copy for yourself
- anticipate any problems in your performance arising from your completed paperwork and collect more information about your performance or related circumstances if relevant
- note down any issues you want to discuss at the appraisal
- review targets in last year's/current PDP – were they met? If not, why not?
- review your personal strengths and areas in need of development
- identify any barriers to your development and possible solutions.

At the appraisal:

- adopt a positive approach to get the most out of your appraisal, putting any apprehension aside and enjoying attention being focused on you and your future plans
- set SMART objectives (*see* Box 2.6): what can you do to improve the service you provide for patients? What personal knowledge and skills do you want/need to improve – and why is the time/cost justified? What do you need to do to stay healthy and well with a good balance to your life?

Box 2.6:   Objectives should be SMART

Specific
Measurable
Agreed
Realistic
Time-related

Activity 2.9: What does appraisal mean to you?

Have a go at describing the meaning below.

-

-

-

-

-

Activity 2.10: How will you benefit from being appraised?

Consider how an appraiser might boost your personal development and performance in your day-to-day work.

-

-

-

-

-

-

References

1 Conlon M (2003) Appraisal: the catalyst of personal development. *BMJ.* **327**: 389–91.

2 Chambers R, Mohanna K, Wakley G and Wall D (2004) *Demonstrating Your Competence 1: healthcare teaching.* Radcliffe Medical Press, Oxford.

3 Wakley G, Chambers R and Field S (2000) *Continuing Professional Development in Primary Care.* Radcliffe Medical Press, Oxford.

4 Nursing and Midwifery Council (2002) *Code of Professional Conduct.* Nursing and Midwifery Council, London.

5 Nursing and Midwifery Council (2001) *The PREP Handbook.* Nursing and Midwifery Council, London.

6 Cooke M (2003) Personal communication.

7 Good Medical Practice (2001) *Good Medical Practice.* General Medical Council, London.

8 www.gpwsi.org

9 Nocon A and Leese B (2004) The role of UK general practitioners with special clinical interests: implications for policy and service delivery. *BJGP.* **54**: 50–6.

10 General Practitioners Committee/The NHS Confederation (2003) *New GMS Contract. Investing in General Practice.* GPC, London.

11 National Institute for Clinical Excellence (NICE), www.nice.org.uk

12 Scottish Intercollegiate Guidance Network (SIGN), www.sign.ac.uk

13 Irvine D and Irvine S (eds) (1991) *Making Sense of Audit.* Radcliffe Medical Press, Oxford (out of print).

14 Department of Health (2003) *EPP Update Newsletter.* DoH, London. *See* Expert Patient Programme on www.ohn.gov.uk/ohn/people/expert.htm

15 Mohanna K and Chambers R (2000) *Risk Matters in Healthcare.* Radcliffe Medical Press, Oxford.

16 Maxwell RJ (1984) Quality assessment in health. *BMJ.* **288**: 1470–2.

17 Honey P and Mumford A (2000) The *Learning Styles Questionnaire 80-item Version.* Peter Honey, Maidenhead.

18 Chambers R (1999) *Survival Skills for GPs.* Radcliffe Medical Press, Oxford.

19 Chambers R, Wakley G, Iqbal Z and Field S (2002) *Prescription for Learning: techniques, games and activities.* Radcliffe Medical Press, Oxford.

20 Chambers R, Schwartz A and Boath E (2003) *Beating Stress in the NHS.* Radcliffe Medical Press, Oxford.

21 Chambers R, Wakley G, Field S and Ellis S (2003) *Appraisal for the Apprehensive.* Radcliffe Medical Press, Oxford.

3

Being an effective appraiser

Appraisers must take their responsibility seriously and prepare well for each appraisal, to do justice to each unique professional conversation. They should keep themselves up to date, not only with the clinical and non-clinical requirements of their own professional role, but also with any developments of the appraisal process in their practice or primary care organisation (PCO) and with any new approach to quality assurance of continuing professional development (CPD).

Being an effective appraiser requires having a good understanding of:

- the positive and developmental nature of appraisal
- how to prepare for an appraisal
- the structure and process of appraisal
- stages in an appraisal discussion
- the timetable in the appraisal process
- possible pitfalls
- ground rules
- the qualities that an effective appraiser should possess
- the scope of appraisal and what distinguishes the role of an appraiser from other work-related roles
- how to overcome problems and constraints that might crop up during an appraisal discussion.

Here are some ideas of what you should be aiming for in the appraisal process with those you are appraising.[1]

- The appraisee and the appraiser need to meet regularly. In the best schemes progress is reviewed frequently. Annual reviews are insufficient.
- Nothing should come as a shock at a formal appraisal interview. Ongoing feedback should be a regular feature in people's everyday work in the NHS.
- Appraisal is not a substitute for day-to-day supervision, support and feedback on performance.
- Appraisers have an ongoing responsibility to ensure that the people they appraise can achieve the agreed objectives and where necessary give or direct them to help.
- The person being appraised plays the major part in setting his or her objectives but these must be set within the overall framework of what staff in that grade are expected to achieve or be able to demonstrate.
- Self-assessment is an important part of appraisal, but the appraiser must curb the tendency of individuals being appraised to be unreasonably self-critical.
- Appraisal interviews are best conducted on a one-to-one basis.

- Any promised level of confidentiality should be respected. The only exception to this is where aspects of poor performance come to light when the appraiser has a professional responsibility to protect patients. This proviso should be made explicit at the start of the appraisal process.

Preparing for the appraisal session as an appraiser[1-3]

It is important that as an appraiser you are at least as well-prepared for each meeting as those you are appraising. It is primarily your responsibility to set out an agenda and guide the meeting. Figure 3.1 may provide you with some structure to help move the meeting forward. Providing a relaxed atmosphere is crucial, but equally it is important not to spend too much time chit-chatting before you move on to the purpose of the appraisal meeting.

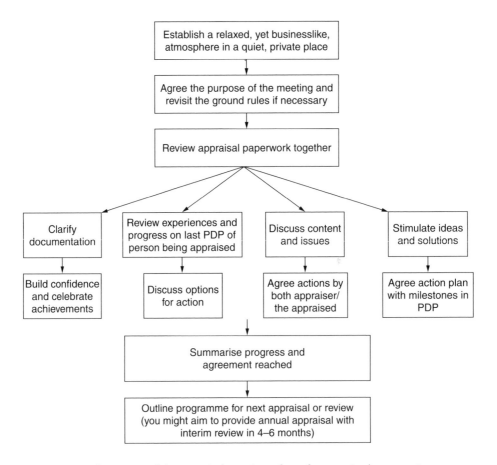

Figure 3.1:   The process of the appraisal meeting – from the appraiser's perspective.

Remember that issues should be explored from the perspectives of the person being appraised and those of your practice, PCO or the NHS as a whole. Keep clarifying what is being said, so that you both share the same perspectives and obtain a full picture. At the end of the meeting it is important that the actions are agreed by both of you.

Box 3.1 gives you a guide on the range of questions you might pose when you review progress from the last appraisal and/or review of someone's personal development plan (PDP).

Box 3.1: Review of progress since previous appraisal and personal development plan agreed

- What did you actually do?
- What had you hoped to achieve?
- What did you actually achieve?
- Did any learning points crop up unexpectedly?
- How would you describe the personal benefits?
- What do you think you could do next to build on your achievements?

Timetable for the appraisal process: countdown as an appraiser

Ongoing

- Know the full details of the way the appraisal process and systems operate in your practice, organisation or trust.
- Know how and when you will undertake appraisal, and how those being appraised will be notified and sent appraisal forms to complete.
- Consider if your training as an appraiser has been sufficient, or if you have learning needs – and if so, address them.

Three weeks before at the latest

- Plan – where the meeting will take place. This should be in a quiet room where you are unlikely to be disturbed. Book a convenient time and private place so that you will not be interrupted. Make sure you have allowed plenty of time for the session and that as far as you can you will be able to be punctual. Set aside at least one hour. Reserve a time when you are both free from other commitments. It cannot be done in the corner of a busy room when you are both busy, with lots of other people listening.
- Communicate with the person you are appraising – give them plenty of warning of the date and time of the meeting, explain what you expect from them and remind them of the purpose of the review.
- Collate paperwork – check you have a copy of the appraisee's job description (if appropriate) and any relevant documentation relating to his or her work or performance. Make sure you have a copy of his or her previous appraisal (if relevant), agreed PDP and any past objectives.

- Gather information – facts and figures on past and recent performance as appropriate, feedback from other individuals with whom the person works by agreement, information on possible development opportunities and training events or sources of support that may be useful. Collect information from: the logbook or portfolio of the person being appraised, examination results or qualifications attained, training or courses attended, reports or presentations given, other colleagues or staff, etc. The proportions of effort both you and those you are appraising put into collating information for appraisal will depend on your local appraisal system and the extent to which you collect subjective and objective information of someone's performance.
- Swap and share all information available to you both – information about someone's performance should not be revealed for the first time by either of you when you come to do the appraisal.

One week before at the latest

- Reflect on the paperwork you have gathered and the contents of the person's completed appraisal form.
- Draw up the meeting structure, describing the tasks and objectives to discuss, and agree with the individual being appraised.

At the appraisal

- Create an informal and relaxed atmosphere and put the person being appraised at ease.
- Explain the purpose and timing of the appraisal meeting and what outcomes you expect.
- Agree the 'ground rules', including any limits set on confidentiality (such as belief that patient safety may be at risk).
- Share your intended agenda and invite the person being appraised to add any issues or items.
- Discuss how you will be taking notes and what will happen to your records.
- Encourage the person being appraised to review his or her performance as you talk through achievements of last year's PDP.
- Let the person being appraised do most of the talking.
- Follow your pre-prepared structure, but be flexible and vary the timing according to the other person's needs.
- Some prompts to reflect on during the appraisal: national and local priorities,[4] review of any significant event analysis, review of audits and protocol developments, review of prescribing data and referral data, working relationships with colleagues, any feedback from or involvement from patients, last year's PDP and goals set there.
- Discuss the person's performance focusing on facts and avoiding subjective judgements. You could structure discussion around the three domains of knowledge, skills and attitudes, or the core competencies of the specialty or discipline or post of the person you are appraising.
- Give feedback by emphasising positives and encouraging him or her to reflect on and value achievements.
- Discuss any areas where his or her performance could have been improved and why – issues may be personal or operational, or relate to the limited availability of resources or training opportunities.

- Discuss possible career paths or first steps and how the person being appraised views them.
- Jointly agree the objectives for a future PDP based on the appraisal discussion (*see* Box 3.2).
- Jointly agree what training and development needs have been identified and encourage the person being appraised to make a realistic plan.
- Summarise what has been agreed – the other person first and you as appraiser afterwards reaffirming, revising or adding. Reinforce their strengths and opportunities, and the ways you have jointly identified for them to resolve problems and address their needs.
- Agree their plan for the future.
- Agree the next steps – the timescale for writing up documentation, an interim review date, the next appraisal date, etc. Some appraisers organise the appraisal session so that they have a short break in which to reflect at the end of the appraisal, then complete paper records and share this report with the person being appraised.

After the appraisal

- Complete paperwork and share a copy with those you have appraised.
- Feed back appraisal information in an anonymous way to the PCO to inform its planning process. It may be that the clinical governance lead in your trust or organisation has a central role in this process, collating appraisal information from all the workforce to inform the organisation's various strategies (*see* Chapter 1).
- Organise an interim review as appropriate – a phone call to check on progress or resolution of issues, a face-to-face meeting for more substantial concerns, etc.

Box 3.2:   Example of employee appraisal objective setting and action planning[5]

Staff appraisal action plans are made up of two key areas.

- Objectives: setting goals and priorities for the coming year linked to the team/department plan and what actions will be taken to achieve them. Objectives should derive from changes occurring in the practice/department, ideas for improvements, changes occurring elsewhere in the trust, things that you know you could do better.
- Personal development plan (PDP): identifying and prioritising appropriate training and development needs and opportunities (linked to the needs of the organisation).

Pitfalls in appraisal

Good planning and preparation, and thoughtful training of the appraiser should increase the likelihood that appraisal will be a positive and developmental experience for the person being appraised. But despite your best efforts things may not go as well as you plan. Box 3.3 describes some of the issues that can arise.

Box 3.3: Possible pitfalls in appraisal

- Poor planning and preparation
- Poor selection or matching of appraiser and those appraised, creating a clash of personalities or renewing previous conflicts
- Role of appraiser not clear, especially if the appraiser has other roles and responsibilities in respect of those he or she is appraising, e.g. line management, educational supervisor
- Too little or too much formality between the appraiser and those being appraised
- Failure to set and measure clear outcomes
- Failure to establish rapport
- Objective setting not appropriate or non-existent
- Lack of time
- No, or confusing, ground rules
- Breach of confidentiality
- Line manager feeling excluded or threatened, if not also acting as appraiser

---

Many of the potential pitfalls of the appraisal process listed in Box 3.3, and more, appear in the report given in Box 3.4 of an appraisal that went badly. Following our guidance about good practice as an appraiser should ensure that no one you appraise has a similar experience.

Box 3.4: Reflections on annual appraisal – a sorry story from a GP after his appraisal[6]

'We shake hands, sit down and immediately I am told to move to a different seat. My appraiser's head is now silhouetted against a bright window, his face in shadow. I feel disadvantaged and dominated before the appraisal has even begun.

During the following three hours my professional and personal life is taken apart meticulously and with surgical precision. The pieces fall to the floor and no attempt is made to form them back into a cohesive whole. I feel naked and dirty as I am examined microscopically for any flaws. Every chink in my armour is probed, all weaknesses exposed: I never knew I had so many.

The appraiser has taken notes, but never once does he open the appraisal folder that took me so many hours to collate. An audit of the appointments system is singled out for criticism: I am told that we should have had a gut feeling about the outcome and need not have carried it out. Turning to his notes, my inquisitor grills me on entries from my learning activity log. He has not recorded dates, so I have to scrabble backwards and forwards through the log frantically trying to find the entries concerned, feeling flustered and foolish.

He jots cursory comments on the forms; the goods and excellents that he writes do not reflect the content of our discussion, but I am too drained to care. The agreed actions are either "nil new" or "no problems" or just left blank. Numbed, I sign my agreement.

continued opposite

We turn to the personal development plan next. I ask my appraiser to sign off my existing plan, which has formed a large part of the appraisal folder, and am stunned when he refuses point-blank to sign off any part of it, dismissing it all as irrelevant. I realise that many more hours of my work have been wasted. He conjures up a new plan for me in just two short sentences. Meekly, like a schoolchild, I write to his dictation.

I was told that appraisals were nothing to worry about, and approached this one without concern. I thought that I was well prepared and that I had documented my appraisal folder well. Instead, the experience was a revelation, a humiliating and humbling experience. I have given much and gained little or nothing. This year's appraisal has robbed me of my confidence, but only just for now, and I intend to get it back. There remains a nagging concern: will I have to go through all this again next year?'

Ground rules

Start by agreeing ground rules for meeting and how or whether you will audiotape your meeting. Clarify the objectives and outcomes that you both want to cover. You may wish to revisit the ground rules from time to time, or at the start of each session, to check that you both continue to be happy with your agreement. The ground rules should cover:

- main purpose and focus of the meetings
- expectations of appraiser and those appraised
- commitment to the appraiser process
- confidentiality and any exceptions – in both a personal and professional capacity
- exiting/opting out
- responsibility for arranging appraisal meetings
- frequency of meetings – any interim reviews expected
- length of appraisal meeting
- documentation/record keeping – what and who is keeping it
- how to evaluate feedback (from those you have appraised)
- personal boundaries
- any potential conflicts of interest and agree action (*see* below).

Confidentiality is a tricky issue. On the one hand the appraiser and those he or she is appraising need to develop a trusting relationship where confidences are welcomed and respected. On the other hand, if patient safety seems to be threatened from another's clinical practice, and that risk persists, a health professional or manager has an ethical obligation to take action to remove that risk to patient safety, and may break confidentiality if there is no other way forward. This potential conflict and any other emanating from other roles of the appraiser and those they are appraising in their respective organisations (e.g. line management or educational supervisor) need to be discussed and the limits of confidentiality agreed as relevant.

Activity 3.1: What ground rules are essential for you in an appraisal session? Have a go at writing them down drawing from the list above.

-

-

-

-

-

-

-

-

-

Qualities of an appraiser

There has been little specific guidance about who should be appointed as appraisers, or what knowledge, skills and experience they should possess at appointment. For the majority of those working in the NHS the appraiser is their line manager, whereas for independent contractors (GPs, pharmacists, optometrists and dentists) who do not have line managers, CPD tutors or a peer/colleague may fill the appraiser role. The Department of Health has clarified the peer nature of appraisal for doctors: 'the appraiser (of a GP) should be another GP, who will have been properly trained in carrying out appraisal' and that 'the senior clinician/clinical governance lead for appraisal co-ordinates the design, implementation and conduct of GP appraisal' in a primary care trust.[7] Training should 'equip appraisers with the skills necessary to carry out appraisal effectively'.[8] The General Practitioners Committee (GPC) has recommended that the GP appraiser should 'normally be actively working in general practice and, ideally, work in the area so that he or she is aware of any local issues or problems. Appraisers should also have the backing of the local profession.'[9] The GPC has warned against clinical governance leads becoming appraisers because of potential conflicts of interest, and has indicated that 'a background in training and development (e.g. be a GP trainer)' may be relevant. No generally agreed job description or person specification for an appraiser has been issued.

Ability to listen is a particularly important skill for an appraiser to have. This means not interrupting, not dominating the conversation, and not going in with pre-judged ideas and conclusions already made. The balance of talking in an appraisal interview should be roughly 80:20 between the person being appraised and the appraiser.

An effective appraiser will:[3]

- use description, not judgement
- keep it friendly, verbally and non-verbally, even if he or she does not like the person
- identify and reinforce strengths
- exactly define and mutually agree on problems
- collect objective evidence
- collaborate on constructive solutions
- identify and use 'carrots' and 'sticks' to make effective change happen
- keep checking: preferably to catch them doing things right
- not capitulate on their 'bottom line', that is, their expectations of consistently good practice from those that they are appraising.

Key skills are summarised in Box 3.5. Chapters 4 and 5 consider the skills an effective appraiser needs in more depth.

Box 3.5:   Key skills that an effective appraiser will possess and use[3]

- Listen
- Reflect back what is being said by those being appraised
- Support
- Treat information in confidence
- Inform without censuring
- Judge constructively
- Identify educational needs
- Construct and negotiate achievable plans

Activity 3.2: What qualities do you think you have to enable you to be an effective appraiser?

-

-

-

-

Distinguish the appraiser role from others you might have

It is vital that you have a clear understanding of your role and responsibilities as an appraiser and know the boundaries between your remit and that of other roles. Table 3.1 clarifies the various characteristics of educational/managerial posts which have overlapping areas.

A mentor is an individual possessing expert knowledge, skill or experience who acts to help the person being mentored to:

- develop and re-examine their own ideas to realise their potential
- be guided on personal, professional and educational matters in a relationship of mutual trust and respect.[10]

A counsellor acts to help people to:

- understand their emotions, abilities, interests and special aptitudes
- make and carry out appropriate life choices and plans and to achieve satisfactory adjustments in life
- acquire information about educational and career opportunities within a changing society.

A coach[11] motivates, encourages and helps an individual to improve his or her skills, knowledge and attitudes in his or her personal and professional lives so that the person:

- is challenged to perform at his or her best
- deepens his or her learning
- enhances his or her quality of life
- focuses on specific objectives within a defined time period.

A preceptor[12] is an experienced individual who provides clinical and professional support to facilitate student learning:

• usually short term
• to enable individuals to develop knowledge and competence after someone has recently qualified, or when someone needs to learn a specific skill
• by supervising, teaching, role modelling and evaluating students – orienting the student to the role at work and monitoring progress.

Preceptorship is usually more intensive than clinical supervision.

A clinical supervisor is an experienced person who supports an individual or group in either the short or long term and:

• aims to develop knowledge and competence, encourage self-assessment and analytical and reflective skills
• enhances consumer protection and safety of care in complex clinical situations.

Table 3.1: Differentiating the *appraiser* from other roles[10]

Role	One-to-one	Group	Long-term	Short-term	Management-led	Personal development	Professional development
	Characteristics of role and responsibilities						
Coach	X			X		X	X
Mentor	X		X			X	X
Preceptor	X			X			X
Assessor	X			X	X		X
Clinical supervisor	X	X	X			X	X
Appraiser	X			X	X		X

Anticipating and overcoming likely barriers in the appraisal discussion

Here is a summary of some of the possible problems that can occur with the appraisal discussion and ideas for solutions. They have been generated from a variety of sources, including experienced appraisers.[13] Some common themes emerge at all levels of experience of appraisers.

Appraisal forms not completed

Solutions

• Appraiser to take time and help those being appraised to fill in the forms. This uses the time and skill, not to mention goodwill of the appraiser. This may be acceptable

in the first year to familiarise individuals with the process, but would probably not be acceptable subsequently.
- PCO sets firm rules and rigorous processes to ensure that only those with completed forms get booked for appraisal.
- Educational sessions run by local appraisers held for those waiting to be appraised to advise and give help with filling in the forms, to introduce the process and explain the forms, and answer queries without actually completing forms.
- If the appraisers themselves run the booking process, the personal touch can ensure that forms are received in time, so that those awaiting appraisal are letting down a local colleague rather than the faceless PCO.

Doing an appraisal where you are not an appropriate appraiser

Solutions
- Having a prior policy on appropriate allocation of appraisers.
- No independent contractor appraisers should appraise their business partners or locums who are extensively used in their own practice.
- Avoid using the same appraiser too often, but also avoid change too often as building a relationship can be very useful.
- There should be an element of choice about the identity of the other, for the appraiser and those to be appraised.

No progress year on year on objectives set in last year's appraisal or PDP. Last year's objectives have still to be achieved in whole or part

Solutions
- Set targets and timescales within the appraisal and document clearly.
- Review regularly until the person being appraised is back on course. Arrange a follow-up call in six months' time for the appraiser to make contact and discuss progress.
- Ensure objectives set in the PDP or at the appraisal are realistic and appropriate.
- Increase understanding of the perspective of the person being appraised. Recognise pressures that healthcare professionals can be under and why they may have failed to deliver.
- Identify 'carrots and sticks' to help ensure that realistic objectives will be achieved.
- Troubleshoot subsequent progress. Keep tabs on the situation and give encouragement.

Conflict of interests

For example, if the appraiser is the 'line manager' of the person being appraised.

Solutions
- Clarify your relationship. If it is impossible to establish sufficient trust, then you need to find a different appraiser/individual match.
- Agree boundaries.
- Develop the right balance between empathy and intimacy.

Criticism of individual being appraised by appraiser
Solutions
- Both should be aware of the sensitivities of individuals being appraised to any criticism and take the utmost care with formal and informal, verbal and non-verbal feedback.
- Discuss problems analytically without bringing personalities into it.
- The appraiser should use a constructive feedback technique (*see* page 70). Being descriptive allows you to assume the role of concerned friend and advisor rather than an outraged colleague or line manager.

Undue sexual attraction between appraiser and those being appraised
Solutions
- Take care to act professionally at all times.

Individuals being appraised have unduly low self-esteem or are self-critical
Solutions
- Appraisers should identify and reinforce strengths.

Problem areas vague and/or multifactorial
Solutions
- Problems need exact definition not generalisations.
- Appraisers should encourage those being appraised to describe facts and plan to collect objective evidence.
- Find constructive solutions. Each specific problem area should have an agreed method of targeted training and objectives to be achieved in specified timescale.
- Appraisers are unyielding in their minimum expectations of good practice (where there are adequate resources).

Non-participation in the appraisal process

Solutions

- Elicit the reasons for this. Often those being appraised have a political agenda or are just worried that the process is really a judgemental assessment.
- Being positive and encouraging from the outset, finding something to praise and working to assure those being appraised that you are 'on the same side'.

Individual being appraised is about to retire, so cannot see the relevance for setting objectives

Solutions

- Help the individual to think about retirement. Sometimes a discussion can make people realise that they do not want to retire completely, merely reduce their hours or do something else with part of their work time.
- Any health professional planning to work privately, or part time after retirement, will still need a licence to practice or to be approved by their regulatory body. Reminding them of this might help participation in appraisal.

Individual being appraised tries to pull seniority

Solutions

- Try to understand their motives as for non-participation from other causes.
- Use the PCO management to explain about the essential nature of appraisal and to back you up.

Appraiser feels intimidated by individual he or she is appraising

Solutions (while maintaining confidentiality)

- Boost appraiser confidence by good-quality training and maybe doing some fairly straightforward appraisals to start with.
- Appraiser support group.
- Appraiser buddy or mentor.
- Email support network.

Getting bogged down in the process of appraisal rather then the content

Solutions

- Good preparation and clarity about what is expected in each section.

- Writing down some key questions beforehand.
- Reading and re-reading the information supplied by those you are appraising to familiarise yourself with the key issues that apply.

Those being appraised 'sabotage' the appraisal discussion

Solutions

- Refuse to be drawn into political discussions about the process.
- Spend time at the start or in a pre-appraisal meeting defining the 'contract' for the meeting.

Pressure of time

Solutions

- Both appraiser and individuals being appraised: assess the time needed realistically and plan for it.
- Define clearly in advance how much time is available and stick to it.

Those being appraised request that other colleagues are present during the appraisal to help provide further information

Solutions

- Contract clearly at the beginning, so that the role of these people is clear and whether they will be present throughout.
- Consider whether they will influence the process and record the influence of others in the appropriate part of the appraisal paperwork.

References

1   Chambers R, Wakley G, Field S and Ellis S (2003) *Appraisal for the Apprehensive.* Radcliffe Medical Press, Oxford.

2   Chambers R, Mohanna K, Wakley G and Wall D (2004) *Demonstrating Your Competence 1: healthcare teaching.* Radcliffe Medical Press, Oxford.

3   Mohanna K, Wall D and Chambers R (2004) *Teaching Made Easy: a manual for health professionals* (2e). Radcliffe Medical Press, Oxford.

4   General Medical Council (2001) *Good Medical Practice.* General Medical Council, London.

5   North Stoke Primary Care Trust (2003) *Appraisal Policy.* North Stoke PCT, Stoke-on-Trent.

6   Archer M (2003) Reflections on annual appraisal. *BJGP.* **53**: 982–3.

7   Department of Health (2002) *NHS Appraisal. Appraisal for General Practitioners Working in the NHS.* Department of Health, London. www.dh.gov.uk/PolicyAndGuidance/Human ResourcesAndTraining/LearningAndPersonalDevelopment/Appraisals/fs/en

8   Leech P (2002) *Future GP Appraiser Training* (letter to chief executives of PCTs). Department of Health, London.

9   General Practitioners Committee (2002) *GP Appraisal. Guidance for GPs.* British Medical Association, London.

10 Bayley H, Chambers R and Donovan C (2004) *The Good Mentoring Toolkit for Healthcare.* Radcliffe Publishing, Oxford.

11 Kersley S (2004) The ABC of change. *BMJ Careers.* **328**: s47.

12 Sachdeva AK (1996) Preceptorship, mentorship and the adult learner in medical and health sciences education. *J Cancer Educ.* **11**: 131–6.

13 Willis M and Penney A (2003) Appraisal for the reluctant. In: K Mohanna (ed.) *Educ Prim Care.* **14(4) Supplement**: 558–61.

4

Developing your competence as an appraiser in communication skills and encouraging others in their professional development

Setting out your knowledge and skills as an appraiser based on the NHS Knowledge and Skills Framework

One way to describe the knowledge and skills you will need for your role and responsibilities as an appraiser is the NHS Knowledge and Skills Framework (KSF).[1] This framework seems to be an appropriate tool for describing the characteristics of any employed post in the NHS and is part of the NHS Agenda for Change initiative.[2] Under Agenda for Change, staff employed by the NHS (excluding doctors, independent contractors and their staff) will be placed in one of eight pay bands depending on the knowledge, responsibility, skills and effort needed for their job. The KSF is intended to be used as part of a structured approach to training, development and review, with the overall aim of improving consistency and quality of services to patients. The six core dimensions and 14 specific dimensions of the KSF are based on what knowledge and skills staff are currently expected to possess. Adopting the KSF will have significant implications for revealing previously unfilled and/or unrecognised training needs for all health professionals, managers and the non-professional workforce.

The KSF can be utilised to describe a competent appraiser in the NHS, whatever the setting or professional group, or seniority of the appraiser with those they are appraising. A literature search of the descriptions of a competent appraiser in the context of doctors found that using the KSF tool broadened the range of knowledge and skills expected of a GP appraiser from others' descriptions. The result of this study was that all six core dimensions of the KSF and five of the other 14 specific dimensions were found to be relevant to the job description of an appraiser, as is captured in Box 4.1.[3]

Each dimension of the KSF is further described in levels. Starting with Level 1, each level describes successively more advanced knowledge and skills, and/or increasing complexity of application of knowledge and skills to the demands of work. The content of each level builds on that of the preceding level. The number of levels in each of the 22 dimensions of the first version of the KSF varies between four and five.[1]

The description of your role and responsibilities as an appraiser, based on the KSF, will allow your primary care organisation (PCO) to undertake performance management of you as an appraiser, as well as facilitating your professional development, as you identify learning needs by comparing your current knowledge and skills with those expected now and in the near future. You might keep a portfolio of your learning and work as an appraiser, showing how you meet the defined levels of knowledge and skills in your job description. You could include a section in your main job description of your roles and responsibilities as an appraiser based on the KSF. This should map easily into your main job description if it, too, is based on the KSF. If you are employed by the NHS, this approach should enable you to clarify with your employer how you are operating as an appraiser over and above your everyday job.

Box 4.1: Descriptions of knowledge and skills of an appraiser organised under the NHS Knowledge and Skills Framework[3]

The first six are core dimensions, and are followed by five specific dimensions.

1 Communication: consistently practise good communication skills with those appraised and your organisation (Level 4)
2 Personal and people development: develop own and others' knowledge and practice across professional and organisational boundaries in relation to appraisal (Level 5)
3 Health, safety and security: promote others' health, safety and security in relation to appraisal (Level 1)
4 Service development: develop and improve NHS service through the appraisal process (Level 3)
5 Quality improvement: demonstrate personal commitment to quality improvement, offering others advice and support as integral part of appraisal process (Level 4)
6 Equality, diversity and rights: enable others to exercise their rights and promote equal opportunities and diversity through appraisal (Level 4)
7 Promotion of self-care and peer support: encourage others to promote their own current and future health and wellbeing through appraisal (Level 1)
8 Ability to manage the appraisal process: process and manage data and information and maintain confidentiality (Level 3)
9 Ability to carry out needs assessment: interpret, appraise and synthesise data and information appropriately within appraisal process (Level 3)
10 Ability to contribute to and/or co-ordinate the support system for the appraisal process: develop and sustain partnership working with those appraised and the practice/primary care organisation/Deanery (appraisers: Level 2; appraiser leads: Level 4)
11 Leadership skills: lead others in the development of knowledge, ideas and work practice as integral part of appraisal process (Level 2)

N.B.: The dimensions of the KSF have been interpreted in the context of appraisal.

The description of the competent appraiser matched against the KSF can be in-corporated into the appraiser's job description (*see* Appendix 1). Being an appraiser can be considered as a stand-alone post, as for instance for appraisers of independent contractors, where peers are employed to undertake appraisal of their fellow GPs, pharmacists, dentists or optometrists. Or the attributes of an appraiser can be incorporated into the job description of his or her main job, as for instance with managers or health professionals employed by an NHS organisation.

You might be able to demonstrate that you are competent as an appraiser by referring to evidence of your knowledge and skills matched against the list of competencies in Box 4.1, but that does not ensure that you perform consistently well. One of the downsides of tools and frameworks such as the NHS KSF is that they imply that performance can be anticipated and measured, whereas in reality in healthcare it is difficult to do so in a complex and changing health setting.

Being competent is the 'ability to perform the tasks and roles required to the expected standard',[4] where knowledge and skills are components of competence. Performing consistently well will depend on your personal application and morale as an appraiser, the availability of resources and support such as training and protected time, and the expectations and preparedness of those being appraised. It is not sufficient to have knowledge and know-how (competence); you also need to apply your knowledge and skills in practice as consistently good performance in action. As an appraiser you need to possess high-order professional judgement as well as the core competencies to be *able to apply* your knowledge and skills consistently in appropriate ways with a range of people you are appraising. As an appraiser you will have many attributes relating to the KSF over and above those described in Box 4.1 to be competent to deal with complex situations that may crop up between you and those you appraise in considering their professional or personal experiences.

We have set out the tools and techniques that will be useful to you as an appraiser for developing your knowledge and skills under the 11 headings of the relevant dimensions of the NHS KSF (*see* Box 4.1). You should read through our descriptions of what each dimension of knowledge and skills might entail. Then consider how your own knowledge and skills match up. If you have a learning need, we offer several alternative ways by which you might build your knowledge and skills or positive attitude for that specific dimension.

This should be useful for your own personal development and appraisal portfolio(s). Various types of audit, feedback from colleagues, peers and those you are appraising, comparison with best practice and critical incident analysis (e.g. a complaint from someone you have appraised) are all good methods of gathering objective evidence – as described in Chapter 2.

This chapter considers how you may develop your competence as an appraiser for the first two dimensions of the NHS KSF: communication and personal and people development. Each section considers the components of the particular dimension of the KSF, and proposes tools and techniques you might use to develop your competence or show others to enable them to improve their performance at work. The remaining nine dimensions from the KSF applicable to appraisers are described in Chapter 5. Subsequently, an approach to demonstrating your competence as an appraiser is covered in Chapter 6, building on the five-staged approach to the evidence cycle, first introduced in Figure 6.1.

The text is interspersed with activities, which should help you to check out how competent you are or reinforce your learning. You might use an activity for your own development or use it to show those you are appraising how to develop knowledge and skills that will help their development or learning.

Dimension 1. Communication: consistently practise good communication skills (Level 4)[1,3]

Effective communication skills

Consistently practise effective communication skills with those you appraise by:

- understanding and applying good interpersonal communication: recognising and taking account of the other's favoured interpersonal style in order to optimise communication between you, and summarising what the person you are appraising says, to check that you are both on the same wavelength
- using active listening
- using supportive, non-verbal body language and reading verbal and non-verbal signals of those you appraise
- establishing rapport with those you appraise and creating a suitable atmosphere to put them at ease
- giving constructive feedback
- recognising and sensitively managing areas of resistance and conflict within the discussion process, managing anger and aggression
- skills: influencing, assertiveness, facilitation
- challenging assumptions and statements of those you are appraising, as appropriate
- enabling a constructive outcome to appraisal to be achieved: judging when further detail is needed, effective summarisation and clarification
- having an enthusiastic and positive attitude to appraisal
- maintaining confidentiality during communication consistent with legislation and NHS policies
- establishing the help that those you appraise require and acting on this appropriately: knowing appraisal system, knowing what the PCO can do to help, identifying resource needs.

Consider the extent to which you:

- have the knowledge and skills
- practise them – during appraisals and in your everyday working life in other aspects of your job (you might generalise to 'colleague or member of staff' in the list above).

Complete your audit checklist in Table 4.1.

How expert are you? Think how expert you are for each aspect of effective communication listed in the left-hand column of Table 4.1.

- Aware? If you are merely 'aware' you might be aware that the particular knowledge and/or skill is important and have undertaken some preliminary reading and learning, but are not yet confident, practised or skilled in employing that feature of effective communication.
- Competent? If you are 'competent' you will have a good basic knowledge and be skilled in communicating with a typical person whom you appraise.
- Expert? If you are an 'expert' you will have an enormous range of experience and intuitive grasp of situations. You will be able to interpret and synthesise information and handle a wide range of communication problems in different contexts.[5]

Table 4.1: Self-check of own knowledge and skills in respect of communication between you as appraiser and those you appraise

Aspect of communication	How expert are you? Aware? Competent? Expert?	How frequently do you use these? At least every day? Weekly? Monthly?
Understand and apply good interpersonal communication, active listening		
Establish rapport with those you appraise		
Use non-verbal body language		
Give constructive feedback		
Recognise and manage conflict		
Challenge other's beliefs constructively		
Skills: influencing, assertiveness, facilitation		
Enable a constructive outcome to appraisal		
Have enthusiastic attitude to appraisal		
Maintain confidentiality		
Establish the help the other person requires		

How frequently do you use that aspect of effective communication? Think how often you employ that feature of effective communication with others at work. Think more widely than appraisal, and of your interactions with colleagues of all levels of seniority and patients. Is it at least daily or at least weekly or at least monthly? The more such knowledge and skills are part of your normal behaviour, the more likely they will feature naturally and consistently in the way you undertake appraisal sessions.

Make your assessment more objective: seek others' views of your competence or performance in relation to effective communication. You might simply ask someone else who knows you well to complete a second copy of the audit Table 4.1 and compare your pre-completed table with their perspective of you – and, of course, discuss any differences with them so that you can learn from their input. You might seek feedback from the person you appraise, or others for whom you have a role or responsibility, such as in line management, educational supervision, mentoring or coaching.

General tips for improving your communication skills[6]

We all think we know about communication skills – and are often baffled when someone misinterprets something we have said or done. No one should be complacent and think they cannot improve their communication skills. You can grade people into being at one of three levels.[7]

1   Unskilled. People at this level use whatever methods come naturally – good or bad. They have little or no insight into the effect their communication has on other people. They tend to blame others for failures or dismiss others as hopeless or incapable of changing.
2   Using acquired tricks. At this level people have learnt some useful communication skills, but they tend to apply them uncritically without observing the effect or noting feedback from others.
3   The skilful communicator has a wide range of appropriate behaviours that can be tailored to the situation and modified according to the feedback received.

You can learn how to observe, evaluate and change how you communicate with other people. Receiving feedback from others helps to make the necessary changes. Understand not just what is said but the feelings behind the words. Consider the verbal and non-verbal aspects of communication, as described in Figure 4.1.

The meaning of language[7–9]

Most of the time we understand what people say, but sometimes our 'wires get crossed'. Some examples of poor language skills are as follows.

- **Taking things literally**. The answer to 'Have you seen that file I put down?' is not 'Yes', but 'It's over there on the table'.
- **Action meanings**. People often use action statements when they do not like to ask for things directly. Saying 'It's very fresh in here with the window open' can be a request for the window to be shut and the speaker will be quite offended if you reply 'Yes, it's nice to have fresh air coming in'.
- **Connotative meanings**. These can suggest emotions but express what is said and what is meant differently. Many people remember their full name being used when someone was telling them off. People who use metaphors implying that the workplace is a war zone (e.g. we will attack this problem on several fronts and defend our position on this matter) may be expressing their inner feelings about it being a battlefield. A reply that is entirely appropriate in a social setting may be regarded as offensive in a work environment (e.g. after someone has spent hours preparing a document, the response should be a proper appreciative message not a scribbled note 'thanks, OK').
- **Using jargon.** The use of jargon can sometimes be an unconscious attempt to prevent communication and understanding – after all if you do not understand what I am talking about you cannot possibly do my job! More often it is the failure to use the feedback (or lack of it) to modify what is being said to the level of understanding of the listener.
- **Using formal or informal styles in the wrong settings**. People speak differently to their friends than to colleagues or to people at work with whom they have an unequal power relationship. You may come across someone using a 'chat-up' style

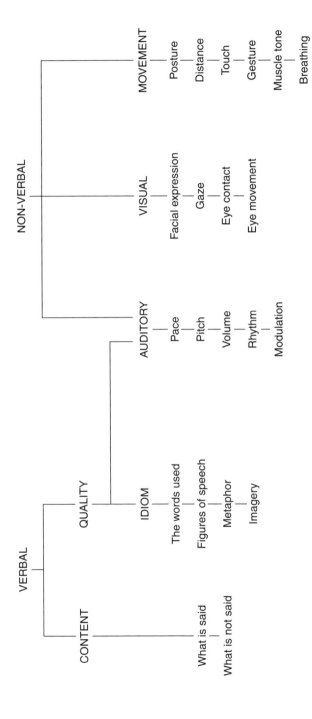

Note: bear in mind that cultural factors may influence what is happening (e.g. the amount of eye contact, gesture or touch may be altered according to the culture of origin or adoption).

Figure 4.1: Signs of the mental state in communication.[6]

with a colleague, or someone introducing their partner as Mr or Mrs Smith at an informal get-together in a pub. Generally, the more formal the event, the more formal the language and some people find it difficult to gauge the right level. Cultural factors affect the situation – what might seem excessively formal to an American may seem over-casual to someone from Japan.

More general tips for improving your skills for good interpersonal communication are given in Box 4.2.

Box 4.2:　Skills for good interpersonal communication[9]

- Listen with genuine interest
- Create a conducive environment
- Be encouraging
- Show understanding and empathy
- Check current understanding
- Reflect/summarise and paraphrase answers
- Use closed questions for exploration
- Use open questions for clarification
- Adopt a similar language and avoid jargon
- Use plural pronouns to indicate partnership
- Be provisional rather than dogmatic
- Be descriptive not judgemental
- Comment on the issues rather than personalities
- Encourage eye contact
- Give information in clear, simple terms and use repetition
- Check understanding
- Use silence

The difference between hearing and listening – use active listening

The quality of attention that you bring to the appraisal session is achieved by a concentrated form of listening. There is a great deal of difference between *hearing* and *listening*. Hearing is a passive activity, while listening is active and requires you to *show* that you have been listening. There is a real difference between the listening that takes place with a patient when taking a case history, and the kind of listening you will need when helping a colleague to reflect on his or her situation. When taking a case history you are assessing what the patient says with a view to making a diagnosis. The first step with those you appraise is to enable them to express themselves fully and feel understood. This process consists of reflecting back what has been said, para-phrasing and summarising at frequent intervals.

Only when someone feels certain that they are understood will they proceed to share their thoughts and feelings. That should help the individuals you are appraising to move forward to thinking about the future and drawing up plans for action.

Exploring

Try to use open questions to expand the conversation that encourage the other person to describe information and explore or reflect on their feelings. Avoid using 'Why?' questions as they tend to trigger defensive responses. Instead, ask 'What?', 'How?' and 'When?' to draw out the person you are appraising.

Creating rapport

Rapport is the process of building and sustaining a relationship of mutual trust and understanding. It is the ability to relate to others in a way that makes people feel at ease. When you have rapport with someone you feel at ease, conversation flows and silences are easy. It is the basis of good communication and is a form of influence. It is a major component of listening, when the whole body indicates interest in what the other person is saying.

Building rapport is a technique described and practised in Neuro-Linguistic Programming (NLP), which is the study of what works in thinking, language and behaviour. You might use NLP to enable those you appraise to plan ahead after identifying their learning and service development needs. NLP is based on a simple model of goal achievement set out as four stages:

- decide what you want
- do something
- notice what happens
- be flexible – be prepared to change.[10]

Steps in creating rapport and relationship building as an appraiser[9]

- You should be aware of yourself and your 'body language'. Make a conscious effort to match or mirror as many of the other person's characteristics as possible: posture and the position of your body, legs, arms, hands and fingers, and how your head and shoulders are held, expression.
- Ensure that you make and keep sufficient eye contact (too much is intimidating).
- Voice – think about the pace, volume and intonation of your voice. Listen to the type of words being used by those you appraise. Try to use a similar voice and words.
- Create an environment that facilitates rapport and easy conversation, for example seating position, dress, décor of room, etc.
- Be friendly and attentive, and adopt an informal style.
- Use plural pronouns to indicate partnership as appropriate, though not to imply that you as the appraiser are taking responsibility for the actions of those you appraise.
- Use self-disclosure about your own fears or experiences to establish trust and common ground (but not too often as the session is focused on the other person's agenda, not yours).
- Make comments that are provisional rather than dogmatic, inviting discussion. Comment on the problem rather than make judgements.
- Ask open rather than closed questions.
- Listen actively and reflectively.
- Pick up and follow themes that those being appraised introduce.

- Use clear, relevant and brief communication rather than rambling anecdotes. It is the other person's agenda that is important in the appraisal session. The appraiser should resist any temptation to indulge him or herself by enjoying reciting his or her own experiences for his or her own benefit.
- Learn to recognise and interpret and use your own feelings so that you do not relay these inappropriately to those being appraised.

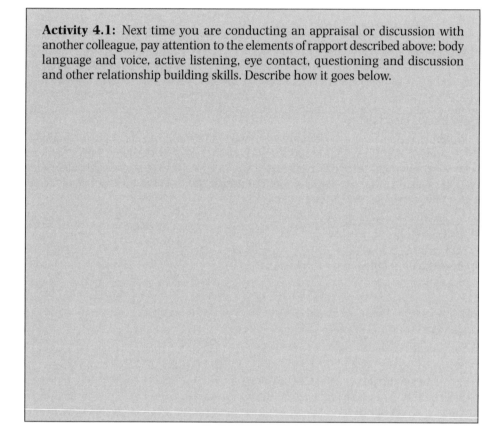

Activity 4.1: Next time you are conducting an appraisal or discussion with another colleague, pay attention to the elements of rapport described above: body language and voice, active listening, eye contact, questioning and discussion and other relationship building skills. Describe how it goes below.

Remembering the JoHari window model

The JoHari window[11] is a useful model for thinking about communication. It will help you to understand the function of feedback and the way you and others relate to each other by interpersonal activity, identifying strengths and learning needs. Figure 4.2 illustrates the concept. The four panes of the 'window' or four quadrants, represent how relationships are built up by an accumulation of information from 'self' and 'others' – in this case you as the appraiser and those you appraise.

Consider the crossed lines that separate the four quadrants as if they can be moved to vary the size of the four quadrants in Figure 4.2 to those of Figure 4.3. The horizontal line represents 'exposure' (that is, extent of self-disclosure by others). By such exposure those being appraised open up, share ideas and information, admit mistakes and talk about their feelings and opinions. As they increase exposure, their

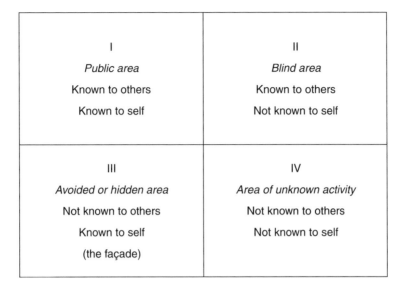

Figure 4.2: JoHari window.

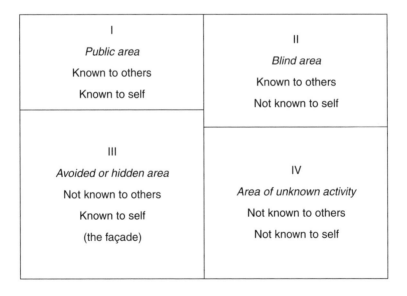

Figure 4.3: JoHari window for new relationships.

'façade' decreases, but the 'blind spot' may increase through less time being given to feedback.

Focusing on giving constructive feedback may increase the façade as it allows less time for 'exposure' for people you appraise to disclose their feelings and fears.

When the appraiser and person being appraised do not know each other very well, the area in quadrant I is small and quadrant III is large, as in Figure 4.3. As an appraiser gets to know the person they are appraising better, quadrant III shrinks in size and quadrant I enlarges. Poor communication between the appraiser and the person they are appraising inhibits the enlargement of quadrant I. The quadrants on the right, especially quadrant II, are susceptible to feedback from you and others, and reducing this area increases the other person's awareness of his or her strengths and learning needs.

Challenge from you or from the colleagues of individuals being appraised, or other external factors, reduces the size of quadrant IV and increases the sizes of quadrants I and II. A person's internal monitoring also helps to reduce the size of quadrant IV, so that their qualities, skills or abilities in this area can become uncovered and recognised, then moved to quadrants I or III.

There is universal curiosity about quadrants III and IV, but this is held in check by custom, social training and fear of what might be revealed. Appraisers need to be sensitive about the covert content of the blind spot, the façade and the hidden area in quadrants II, III and IV, and respect each others' privacy about information kept hidden for reasons of social training or custom. Up to a point, the larger the area called the arena in the top left quadrant in Figure 4.3, the more productive the relationship is likely to be.

You might categorise individuals you appraise into one of four *types* of people using the following Johari window model.

- **Type A**: little exposure, little feedback seeking. These type of people are often perceived as withdrawn, aloof or impersonal, where the unknown square (in Figure 4.2 or 4.3) is the largest. This may induce resentment in others who may take the behaviour personally. It is common in large bureaucratic organisations.
- **Type B**: increased feedback seeking, little exposure. These people decrease the information about themselves available to others, while requiring more from others, either through fear or a wish for power or control. Others may react by withdrawing trust or becoming hostile.
- **Type C**: increased exposure, neglect of feedback. These people are oblivious to the impact they have on others. They have a large blind spot as the opportunity for feedback is rare. They may be confident of their own opinions and insensitive, with little concern for the feelings of others. Listeners may become angry and reluctant to tell them anything.
- **Type D**: balanced. These people have a large arena, as feedback seeking and exposure behaviours are well used. They are open and candid. Initially others may be put on the defensive but once these people are seen as genuine, productive relationships can follow. They induce an open, balanced response in others.

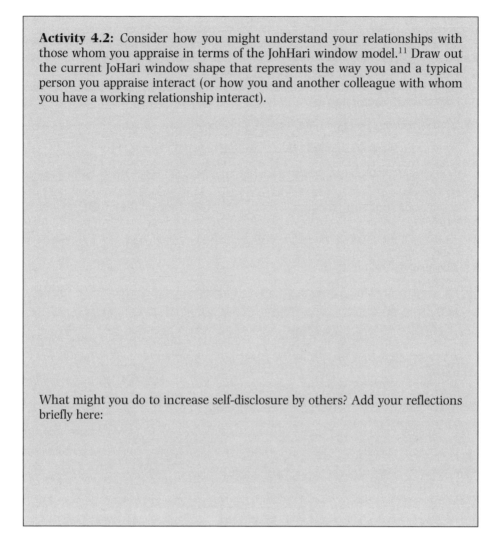

Activity 4.2: Consider how you might understand your relationships with those whom you appraise in terms of the JohHari window model.[11] Draw out the current JoHari window shape that represents the way you and a typical person you appraise interact (or how you and another colleague with whom you have a working relationship interact).

What might you do to increase self-disclosure by others? Add your reflections briefly here:

Building trust and relationships

Trust requires two things: competency and caring. Competency alone or caring by itself will not create trust. Scholtes[12] believes that if you think someone is competent, but you do not think that they care about you or the things that are important to you, you will respect them but not necessarily trust them. On the other hand, if you think someone cares about you but you do not feel they are competent or capable, you will have affection for that person but not necessarily trust them to do the job in hand.

You can encourage people to trust you if you:

- do what you say you will do and do not make promises you cannot or will not keep
- listen to people carefully and tell them what you think they are saying. People trust others when they believe that they understand them
- understand what matters to people. People trust those who they believe are looking out for their best interests.

You can encourage good relationships with people if you:

- are able to talk to each other and are willing to listen to each other
- respect each other and show this in ways that the other person wants
- know each other well enough to understand and respect the other person's values and beliefs
- do not hide your shortcomings. This may improve your image but does not build trust
- do not confuse trustworthiness with friendship. Trust does not automatically come with friendship
- tell the truth! Be honest.

Activity 4.3: Reflect on the extent of the trust there is between you and a typical person you appraise (or another colleague if you have not started appraising yet). What has led to that trust being created? What have you done to create or sustain that trust? List your behaviour and actions or omissions below.

- How I have behaved:

- How person appraised behaved:

Giving constructive feedback[13]

Constructive feedback is the art of holding conversations with others about their performance, and it has two elements: it should contain enough specific detail and advice to enable the recipient to reflect and enhance their practice, and it should be positive and supportive in tone. Effective feedback has an impact not only on the learning process, but also gives messages to others about their effectiveness and worth, and contributes to building their self-esteem.

It is important that as well as being positive in tone, you should balance your commentary between areas to improve and feedback that is positive in content. You should aim to give feedback about their apparent deficiencies *and* strengths. To see why this is so, consider the following model of the development of expertise in Figure 4.4.

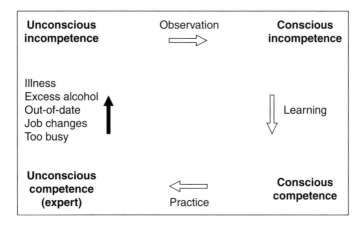

Figure 4.4: The development of expertise (competency cycle).

Starting in the top left-hand quadrant in Figure 4.4, you are blissfully unaware of your shortcomings until something happens to make you aware of them. That might be the realisation when you start working with patients that the education you received at university or college was not appropriate and that you are out of your depth. It could be a patient complaint or adverse incident, or it could be feedback from a teacher or colleague.

This realisation is a painful process, often referred to as cognitive dissonance, but until you become aware you cannot start the process of learning. Remember, it is when you feel uncomfortable that you are just about to learn something. Too much discomfort, however, can be demotivating and some people might give up at this stage if they feel there is too much to learn or they will never be good enough. Some feedback about their other strengths would be supportive at this stage.

The process of learning, with all that that entails, can then proceed and you will master the new understanding, knowledge or task. You reach a stage where you know something new or know how to do something and can perform competently, so long as circumstances remain constant – as represented by the bottom right quadrant of Figure 4.4. With practice and experience you then become expert. You can apply and modify your knowledge and skills in new situations that you may never have met before. At this stage, the bottom left quadrant, you could teach others. It is also the stage when, through familiarity, you can lose sight of your strengths as your skills become automatic. Feedback on performance at this stage needs to include things you are good at so that you do not accept them as commonplace, you can reflect on them, keep them up to date and highlight them. In some ways feedback needs to take you from left to right across the bottom of the competency cycle to make you aware of your expertise again so that you can effectively teach others.

It is possible to move back to unconscious incompetence from the position of expertise, in the direction of the bold arrow, through dementing illness for example, or degenerative disease without insight, or even failure to keep up to date. Feedback in this position is very likely to be difficult – another good reason to include a reminder of remaining skills and positive attributes. (This model has some similarities with the JoHari window – *see* Figures 4.2 and 4.3, which describes balanced communication between feedback seeking and self-disclosure to minimise either the areas of hidden information in a relationship or lack of insight.)

This model provides a theoretical reason behind the observations that constructive feedback needs to contain a commentary on strengths as well as things that need to be improved. It also reinforces the imperative for feedback to 'have teeth'. The skill of the effective appraiser is to find the balance between support and challenge, and the best feedback is high on both support and challenge. Figure 4.5 describes the qualities of feedback of different dimensions.

High support

'That was great, you're obviously trying hard'	'A good effort. I could see how you were drawing the feelings out – I wonder if you got to the crux of the matter?'
Safe, general, potentially patronising	Focused, attentive, potentially threatening

Low challenge | **High challenge**

'Good. Carry on. Seems to be working'	'Well that could have been better – why did you not focus more early on?'
In passing, nothing specific, dismissive	Critical, induces defensiveness, potentially paralysing

Low support

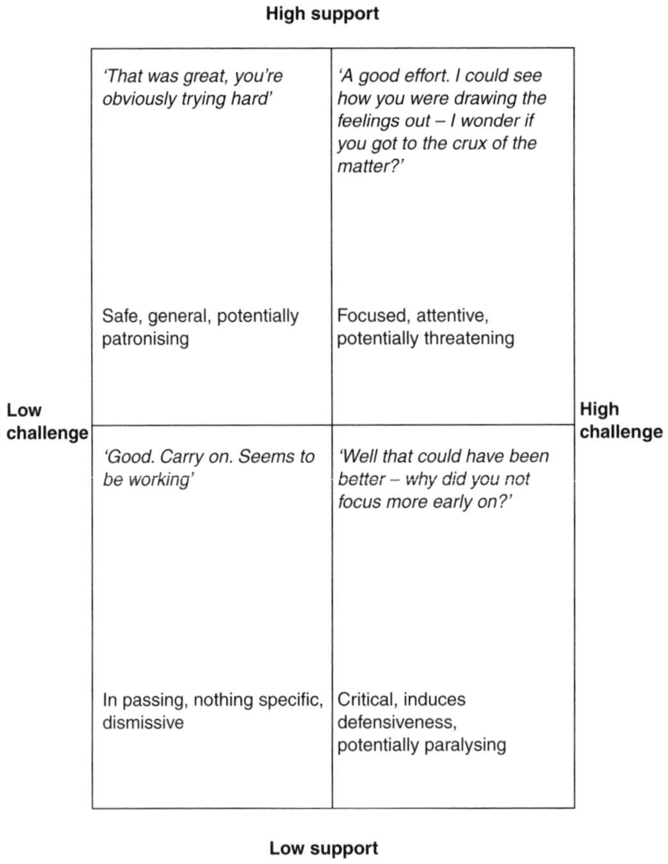

Figure 4.5: The qualities of feedback of different dimensions.

There is one golden rule for giving constructive feedback: give positive praise of things that have been well done first. Some general rules are:

1   focus on behaviour rather than interpretation
2   give specific examples
3   aim to be descriptive or sensory-based rather then interpretive, non-sensory-based
4   aim to be non-judgemental rather then evaluative.

Box 4.3 gives an example of this approach. You can read up elsewhere on different models of giving feedback.[13]

Box 4.3:   An example of a tutorial about a patient case where a preceptor is advising a student nurse

Evaluative, interpretive or judgemental	Descriptive, sensory-based
The beginning was awful, you just seemed to ignore her	At the start you were looking at the notes, which prevented eye contact
The beginning was excellent, great stuff	At the beginning you gave her your full attention and never lost eye contact – your facial expression registered interest in what she was saying
It's no good getting embarrassed when patients talk about their sexual history	I noticed you were very flushed when she spoke about her husband's impotence, and you lost eye contact ...

Activity 4.4: Obtain feedback from colleagues or others to whom you have given feedback recently on their perceptions of the quality of your own feedback. You could ask them to tell you specifically if you obey the general rules for giving good feedback listed above. Try to obtain such feedback from at least three sources.

*   Reflect on the feedback that you have heard and what you can learn about your skills in giving feedback to others.

continued overleaf

- Compare the ways in which these others have given you feedback – what made you feel good and worked well in realising your strengths and deficiencies in the way that feedback was conveyed?

- What aspects of their feedback reports made you feel bad or triggered feelings of defensiveness or worthlessness?

Managing conflict

Conflict and communication are inseparable. Communication can cause conflict: it is a way to express conflict and it is a way to either resolve it or perpetuate it. It is very often a breakdown in communication, or interpretation of that communication, that will inflame the conflict situation. It is the way in which conflicts surface and are addressed or resolved that dictate the outcome.

Conflict is part of change and improvement in the NHS and cannot be avoided. But it can be managed and it can turn out to be positive. Generally, conflicts have two elements, the relationship between the people involved and the issue which is the basis of the disagreement.

As an appraiser, you should be able to intervene effectively in the early stages of conflict between you and anyone you are appraising by preventing, containing or handling it. And you should be able to discuss with them how they should behave in any conflicts in which they are involved in the course of their work.

Techniques for resolving conflict[14] include the following.

1 Acknowledge that conflict exists. The disagreement may be fundamental to an issue or one small component.
2 Recognise potential benefits from the conflict situation: increased understanding and respect for others, exchange of views and attitudes, feelings surfacing, expression of energy and motivation, self-awareness, creativity, novel approaches, opportunities for change, full extent of diversity revealed.
3 Consider the options for handling conflict. For example, compromise, collaboration, co-operation, accommodation.
4 Distinguish between interests and positions within the conflict. This will enable you to understand why different parties disagree and reveal underlying assumptions contributing to the conflict.
5 Try using 'and' instead of 'or'. This approach may enable you to realise that the conflict is not necessary and the seemingly 'conflicting' issues or approaches can be run together quite harmoniously.

6 Acknowledge and face up to 'cultural' differences if the conflict has its roots in deeply held values, beliefs and attitudes. Try to understand other people's perspectives and look at the situation from their viewpoint.

7 Realise that a negotiated settlement is preferable to an unresolved argument.

8 Encourage dialogue, encouraging both sides to suspend judgement while issues are discussed from all perspectives. Keep to facts rather than opinions, seek and explain differences, view complex problems in new ways.

9 Establish 'rules' for conversation and discussion where the speaker may talk without you or others attacking or judging them. Termed 'no cross-talk' it means someone being able to share their experiences, feelings, opinions and hopes on a topic without referring to or reacting to anyone else's contribution and without evaluating what has been said.

Box 4.4 gives a checklist that may be useful at any stage of a conflict situation.

Box 4.4: Tips for handling situations of conflict[13,14]

Do
- cool down the debate in a hot conflict
- convince those involved in conflict that something can be done
- ensure that issues are outlined fully
- acknowledge emotions and different styles
- ensure a comfortable environment for any meeting
- set a timeframe for the discussion
- create good rapport
- use names and, if appropriate, titles throughout the discussion

Do not
- conduct your conversations in a public place
- leave the discussion without an ending – instead create an action plan
- finish other people's sentence for them
- use jargon
- constantly interrupt
- do something else while trying to listen
- distort the truth
- use inappropriate humour

The main thing is to acknowledge and address any conflict and not to avoid it. Describe the issues involved, talk about them and work through the conflict.

Activity 4.5: Think about a conflict situation involving you and another person, and reflect:

- What was the cause of the conflict?

continued overleaf

- How did you respond and what was the impact of this?

- How did the other person respond?

If there was a positive resolution to the conflict, how was this achieved and what did you learn from this that you might apply to how you relate with those you are appraising?

Reflecting on what you have just written and the approaches presented in the text, what could you have done differently to avoid or minimise the conflict or speed its resolution?

Dimension 2. Personal and people development: develop own and others' knowledge and practice across professional and organisational boundaries in relation to appraisal (Level 5)

Effective personal and people development

This means developing your own and others' knowledge and practice across professional and organisational boundaries by:

- understanding the healthcare context relevant to those you are appraising and making realistic allowances for problems and issues (including your and their attitudes, beliefs, learning styles, motivation, etc.) that might obstruct either of you applying best practice
- responding knowledgeably to competing demands within your everyday work
- understanding national and local healthcare priorities and how these are relevant to your circumstances and that of those you appraise

- evaluating the currency and sufficiency of your own knowledge and practice in your everyday work
- applying your own learning to future development of work, arising from undertaking your personal development plan (PDP)
- being able to recognise and acknowledge whether learning has occurred and been applied since the previous meeting, and whether it has addressed the needs of the person concerned
- identifying when local developments and thinking may benefit the practice of others
- working with others (including those you are appraising) to develop, identify and implement appropriate learning opportunities within and outside work
- striving to improve learning strategies and opportunities to increase the overall learning and development of others
- negotiating and encouraging goal-setting and action plans with those you appraise
- supporting the development of a learning and development culture which encourages the sharing of good practice.

Consider the extent to which you:

- have the knowledge and skills
- practise them – in your relationships with those you appraise and in your everyday working life in other aspects of your job (you might generalise to 'colleague or member of staff' in the list above).

Complete your audit checklist below in Table 4.2.

How expert are you? Think how expert you are for each aspect of effective personal and people development that we have listed below in the left-hand column of Table 4.2.

- Aware? If you are merely 'aware', you might be aware that the particular knowledge and/or skill is important and have undertaken some preliminary reading and learning, but are not yet confident, practised or skilled in employing that feature of effective personal and people development.
- Competent? If you are 'competent' you will have a good basic knowledge and be skilled in your own personal development and in developing others as part of the appraisal process.
- Expert? If you are an 'expert' you will have an enormous range of experience and intuitive grasp of situations. You will be able to interpret and synthesise information and handle a wide range of aspects of personal and people development in different contexts.[5]

How frequently do you use that aspect of effective personal and people development? Think how often you employ that feature of effective development with others at work. Is it at least daily or at least weekly or at least monthly? The more such knowledge and skills are part of your normal behaviour, the more likely they will feature naturally and consistently when you meet up with those you are appraising.

Make your assessment more objective: seek others' views of your competence or performance. You might simply ask someone else who knows you well to complete the audit Table 4.2 and compare your pre-completed table with their perspective of you – and, of course, discuss any differences with them so that you can learn from their input. You might seek feedback from people you appraise or others for whom you

Table 4.2: Self-check of own knowledge and skills in respect of personal and people development

Aspect of personal and people development	How expert are you? Aware? Competent? Expert?	How frequently do you use these? At least every day? Weekly? Monthly?
Understand healthcare context relevant to you and others		
Respond to competing demands		
Understand healthcare priorities		
Evaluate own knowledge and practice		
Apply own learning arising from PDP		
Recognise what others have learnt and achieved		
Identify when developments may benefit others		
Work with others to implement learning		
Strive to improve learning strategies and opportunities for others		
Negotiate goal setting, action planning, etc.		
Support development of learning culture		

have a role or responsibility, such as in line management, educational supervision, mentoring or coaching, or as local appraisal lead.

Reflect on your own personal development or that of those you appraise

Understanding the healthcare context and priorities

One of the aims of the appraisal process is to enable others to be more effective in their roles within the NHS. So you need to be familiar with the main strategies driving developments nationally and the local delivery plan of your trust. Find out more about any professional requirements of individuals you appraise from their Royal Colleges or other professional bodies.

Personal learning inventory

Everyone working in the NHS should have a PDP that they review with their manager or another colleague at least annually, probably at their appraisal. So you might evaluate your own knowledge and practice, and reflect on how you have applied what you have learnt in the last year at that review. You might use a personal learning inventory to reinforce your learning and reflect on your continuing professional development (CPD), what you have achieved and what you plan to learn about in the future.

Activity 4.6: Complete your personal learning inventory[15]

1   How will your recent learning influence your approach to:

- lifelong learning?

- professional development?

- personal development?

2   How closely does your own approach to learning match with what is known to herald successful learning:[13]

- based on what is already known
- led by your identified learning/service development needs
- involving your active participation
- using your own resources
- including relevant and timely feedback
- including self-assessment?

3   How will your recent learning influence your leadership and/or management of others?

4   What are the most significant things you have learned from the issues explored in the period you are reviewing?

5   How will what you have learned change your behaviour?

continued overleaf

6 What do you want to do differently in your current role?

7 How have you balanced competing demands?

8 Have you identified how what you have learnt and applied may benefit others? Describe your revised personal learning plan.

Force-field analysis[6]

Using a force-field analysis approach helps people to identify and focus on the positive and negative forces in their work and/or home lives and to gain an overview of the relative weighting of these factors. The exercise is suitable for anyone and everyone at any stage in their career. You might use it to review your current work situation or you might show those you are appraising how to review their own circumstances and need for development.

You should draw a horizontal or vertical line in the middle of a sheet of paper, or show others how to do so. Label one side 'positive' and the other side 'negative'. You/they should then draw arrows to represent individual positive drivers that motivate you/them on one side of the line, and negative factors that demotivate you/them on the other side of the line. The chunkiness and length of the arrows should represent the extent of the influence; that is, a short, narrow arrow will indicate that the positive or negative factor has a minor influence and a long, wide arrow a major effect (*see* Figure 4.6).

Then take an overview of the force-field and consider if you/they are content with things as they are, or can think of ways to boost the positive side and minimise the negative factors. Do this part of the exercise on your/their own, or with a peer from elsewhere.

The analysis exercise helps people to realise to what extent a known influence in their life is a positive or negative factor. For instance they may have assumed that money in the form of a good salary was a positive motivator. But on reflection, they may realise that really, the wish to sustain or increase their income was a negative force on their job satisfaction due to their inability to spend time on meaningful, non-pecuniary activities.

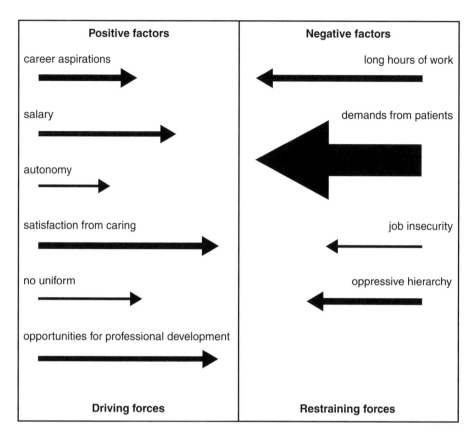

Figure 4.6:   Example of a force-field diagram. Satisfaction with current post as a health professional.

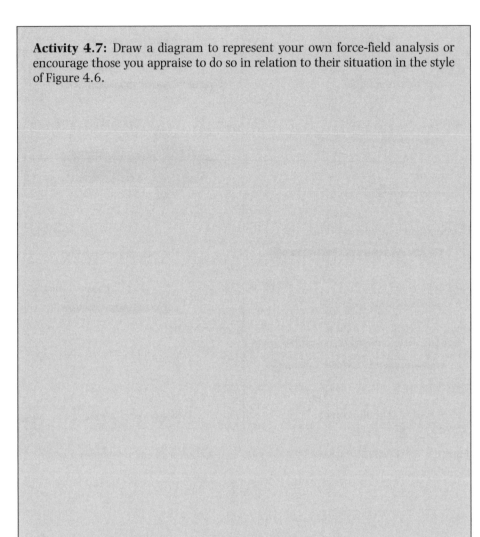

Activity 4.7: Draw a diagram to represent your own force-field analysis or encourage those you appraise to do so in relation to their situation in the style of Figure 4.6.

The next step is for you/them to make a personal or organisational action plan to create the situations and opportunities to boost the positive factors in your/ their life and minimise arrows on the negative side. You or others could invite someone who knows them well to review the force-field analysis they have drawn and let them know honestly of any blind spots and if they have the positive and negative influences in proportion. They can then determine how their needs and priorities should be addressed in planning for the change. This can be done through:

- changing the strength of a driving force: width and length of the arrows
- changing the direction of a force: switching a force to be positive rather than restraining
- withdrawing or minimising a restraining force
- adding or enlarging helping, positive forces.

Bridging the gap[16]

As an appraiser you should help people you appraise to confront the gap between: 'Where they are now' and 'Where they want to be'.

This 'gap' is central to a planned programme of personal development and change, the nature of which depends on the various gaps identified and the person's future goals. This is a model you might use for yourself as an appraiser or NHS professional in your other work; or you might show others as a way of helping them to confront what gaps need to be filled on the path to attaining their goals.

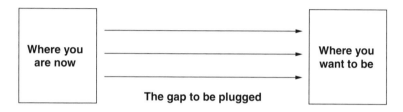

Figure 4.7: An outline gap analysis.

Activity 4.8: Work out your own gap analysis.

1   *Where you are now*: this will include a description of the important aspects of your work/home situation that are relevant to the goals you envisage and changes you want to make. It may cover your strengths and weaknesses in your current role, your experience, your transferable skills, and a review of how your current post measures up to your expectations and values.

2   *Define your future goals*: be as specific as you can be about what you want to achieve. Describe your interests, areas of work and development you'd like to be responsible for or involved in, setting you wish to work in or type of role. Outline your aspirations and preferences.

3   *Describe the gap*: compare items 1 and 2 and describe the main differences between your current state and your desired future position. Make a plan for change with timescales and milestones, so that you can monitor progress. Discuss your plan with others who know you for a reality check. Outline the opportunities that might link where you are now with your future goals.

Change[6,13]

There are lots of reasons why you or those you appraise may be hesitant about changing the way they do things. People underestimate the barriers and hurdles to be overcome before change will be made and sustained. Many of the barriers[17] are listed below.

- Lack of perception of the relevance of proposed change.
- Lack of resources to make change.
- Short-term outlook.
- Conflicting priorities.
- Lack of necessary skills.
- Limited evidence of effectiveness of proposed change.
- Perverse incentives.
- Intensity of personal contribution required.
- Having a poor appreciation of the need to change or considering the need to change to be secondary to other issues.
- Having a poor understanding of the proposed solutions or considering the solution to be inappropriate.
- Disagreeing how the change should be implemented.
- Embarrassment about admitting that what you are doing could be improved.

Change will not be possible unless people are committed to the change and prepared to alter the environment so that it is possible to make the change happen in practice.

As an appraiser you need to understand how people react to change. As Figure 4.8 illustrates, people start off being taken by surprise about a change, even if they anticipate it. There is still a shock element when it first happens and you may not be quite sure what has happened. You move from that shock to pretending it is not going to happen.[6]

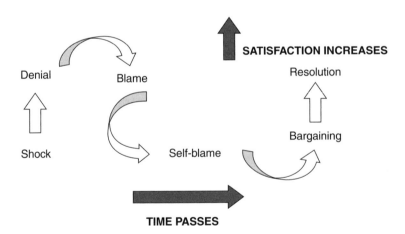

Figure 4.8: Stages in the response to change.

After the denial phase in the change process you move on to find somebody to blame for what has happened – and you tend to blame the messengers who announce the change. After the blame comes self-blame. Part of the next stage, the bargaining, is negotiating that if you do it *this* way they are going to be able to do *that*. Eventually you arrive at the resolution phase where you have accepted the change.

People pass through these different stages of change according to how they are as individuals. When change is imposed, you are very much more resistant and move more slowly. If the effect of the change is serious, your feelings about it will be stronger and you will spend longer in the phases of denial, blame and self-blame.

You need to help others to face up to change by identifying the causes for dissatisfaction with the present situation to have a clear idea of where they are heading. They should map out how to reach their targets, then find their way, in staged steps, to measure the progress towards the target.

Teach them to recognise the roles that people play in response to change.

- The rebel – 'I don't see why I should'.
- The victim – 'I suppose you will make me, but I will drag my feet'.
- The oppressor – 'You all have to do it'.
- The rescuer – 'I will save you all from this terrible change'.

Tips for making changes

It might help to give those you appraise a checklist for planning change that they can adapt to their particular situation.

- Have realistic timescales and be flexible.
- Provide clear communication about what is happening.
- Consult with all the staff, identifying all the problems as they occur.
- Plan for more resources and time than you expect to use.
- Fix interval markers of progress.
- Feed the information back to people about what is happening.
- Identify the anxieties and try to resolve them.
- Consider the effects of this change on other services and people.
- Beware of too many changes taking place at once.
- Recognise that change can be hijacked by vested interests and the direction altered.
- Be prepared to change direction if necessary.
- Beware of a lack of commitment from others.

References

1 Department of Health (2003) *The NHS Knowledge and Skills Framework (NHS KSF) and Development Review Guidance – Working Draft. Version 6.* Department of Health, London.

2 Department of Health (2003) *Agenda for Change. Proposed Agreement.* Department of Health, London.

3 Chambers R, See S, Tavabie A and Hughes S (2004) Composing a competency based job description for general practice appraisers using the NHS Knowledge and Skills Framework. *Educ Prim Care.* **15**: 15–29.

4   Eraut M and du Boulay B (2002) *Developing the Attributes of Medical Professional Judgement and Competence.* University of Sussex, Sussex. Reproduced at www.informatics.sussex.ac. uk/users/bend/doh

5   Benner P (1984) *From Novice to Expert.* Addison-Wesley, London.

6   Chambers R, Wakley G, Iqbal Z and Field S (2002) *Prescription for Learning: techniques, games and activities.* Radcliffe Medical Press, Oxford.

7   Reid M and Hammersley R (2000) *Communicating Successfully in Groups.* Routledge, London.

8   Hargie ODW (1997) *The Handbook of Communication Skills* (2e). Routledge, London.

9   Tate P (2000) *The Doctors' Communication Handbook* (3e). Radcliffe Medical Press, Oxford.

10 Alder H (1996) *NLP for Managers. How to Achieve Excellence at Work.* Piatkus, London.

11 Luft J (1970) *Group Processes: an introduction to group dynamics* (2e). National Press Books, Palo Alto, California.

12 Scholtes P (1998) *The Leaders Handbook: making things happen, getting things done.* McGraw Hill, Maidenhead.

13 Mohanna K, Wall D and Chambers R (2004) *Teaching Made Easy. A manual for health professionals* (2e). Radcliffe Medical Press, Oxford.

14 Elwyn G, Greenhalgh T, MacFarlane F and Koppel S (2001) *Groups: a guide to small group work in healthcare, management, education and research.* Radcliffe Medical Press, Oxford.

15 Garcarz W, Chambers R and Ellis S (2003) *Make Your Healthcare Organisation a Learning Organisation.* Radcliffe Medical Press, Oxford.

16 Bayley H, Chambers R and Donovan C (2004) *The Good Mentoring Toolkit for Healthcare.* Radcliffe Publishing, Oxford.

17 Dunning M, Abi-Aad G, Gilbert D *et al.* (1998) *Turning Evidence into Everyday Practice.* King's Fund, London.

5

Developing your competence as an appraiser in enabling others to perform well and improve their delivery of healthcare

This chapter considers how you may develop your competence as an appraiser in the other nine dimensions of the NHS Knowledge and Skills Framework (KSF).[1] As in Chapter 4, each section considers the components of the particular dimension of the KSF, and proposes tools and techniques you might use to develop your competence or show those you are appraising to enable them to improve their performance at work.

Dimension 3. Health, safety and security: promote others' health, safety and security in relation to appraisal (Level 1)

Health and safety and risk management is about promoting your and others' health, safety and security by:

- being familiar with resources to which you can signpost a person you are appraising for help or advice, e.g. occupational health, stress, financial or relationship difficulties, both within and outside the NHS
- assisting in maintaining a safe working environment. Help those you appraise to identify risks in relation to their health, safety and security or those of their employees
- understanding and reporting any issues or serious concerns throughout the appraisal process that could affect patient care, with explicit consent of those you appraise; without consent if patient safety seems to be at risk
- being clear what constitutes appraisal and what is outside the scope of an appraiser in respect of health or counselling issues
- being confident of and abiding by agreed ground rules for the appraisal system.

Consider the extent to which you:

- have the knowledge and skills
- practise them – in your relationship with individuals you appraise and in your every-day working life in other aspects of your job (you might generalise to 'colleague' or 'member of staff' in the list above).

Complete your audit checklist in Table 5.1.

Table 5.1: Self-check of own knowledge and skills in respect of maintaining health, safety and security

Aspect of health, safety and security	How expert are you? Aware? Competent? Expert?	How frequently do you use these? At least every day? Weekly? Monthly?
Familiar with network to signpost other for help		
Assist in maintaining safe work environment for others		
Understand and report issues that put patient safety at risk		
Be clear what constitutes appraisal; and the boundaries		
Know and abide by agreed ground rules		

How expert are you? Think how expert you are in assisting in maintaining aspects of other's health, safety and security listed in the left-hand column of Table 5.1.

- Aware? If you are merely 'aware' you might be aware that the particular knowledge and/or skill is important and have undertaken some preliminary reading and learning, but are not yet confident, practised or skilled in employing that feature in assisting health, safety and security.
- Competent? If you are 'competent' you will have a good basic knowledge and be skilled in assisting with others' health, safety and security in a typical appraisal.
- Expert? If you are an 'expert' you will have an enormous range of experience and intuitive grasp of situations. You will be able to interpret and synthesise information and handle a wide range of problems in assisting with others' health, safety and security in different contexts.[2]

How frequently do you use that aspect to maintain health, safety and security? Think how often you employ that feature with others at work. Is it at least daily or at least weekly or at least monthly? The more such knowledge and skills are part of your normal behaviour, the more likely they will feature naturally and consistently when you meet up with people you appraise.

Make your assessment more objective: seek others' views of your competence or performance. You might simply ask someone else who knows you well to complete the audit Table 5.1 and compare your pre-completed table with their perspective of you – and, of course, discuss any differences with them so that you can learn from their input. You might seek feedback from those you appraise or others for whom you have a role or responsibility, such as in line management, educational supervision, mentoring or coaching, or as a local appraisal lead.

Signposting individuals to other resources as part of appraisal

If you are to sustain your role as appraiser without moving into other roles, such as counsellor, mentor, educational supervisor or providing pastoral support, you need to be familiar with what local resources there are within and outside the NHS and know how others may access them. Compile a logbook of resources, access arrangements and contact details, local protocols covering the following.

- Occupational health support; for ill and distressed individuals, those with alcohol or drug misuse problems, those whose physical or mental disabilities create functional problems.
- Local process for poor or underperformance of person you are appraising or for them to use if they are concerned about their colleagues.
- Stress management help.
- Explicit protocols for informing others when appraiser suspects or perceives that patient safety is at risk according to whether those whom you appraise do or do not continue to work.
- Processes and resources for providing educational support for general or specific learning and development needs that are or are not recognised by those you appraise.
- System for allocation of resources to help those you are appraising to address their identified learning needs relating to NHS priorities, such as service development and delivery of care – what is available and contact details.
- Advice on financial difficulties.
- Counselling for relationship difficulties, within and outside work setting.
- Career information, guidance and counselling.
- Nature and frequency of ongoing support for training and development, and peer support for appraisers.
- Guarantee of indemnity for appraiser in the unlikely event that an individual you have appraised makes an official complaint: information about explicit limits of indemnity.
- Complaints system for those who have been appraised – nature, how to access, etc.
- Troubleshooting guide: someone or sources of help to consult if problems arise – relating to any/all of above.

Minimise stress and create safe working environment[3]

Stress can be either positive or negative, depending on how you perceive it and how you react to it. If individuals you appraise view sources of stress such as new regulations as challenges rather than burdens, they will probably find ways of managing changes to their advantage with opportunities for learning and growth. *See* Chapter 2, page 29 for more ideas on combating stress.

Health professionals appear to be at higher risk of work-related violence (including woundings, common assault, robbery and snatch theft) than the general population. Practice and community nurses, doctors and other healthcare staff who visit patients in their own homes are often unaware of danger, because their caring nature and their role as the patient's advocate makes them relatively unsuspicious of danger.

The best way to reduce stress caused by aggression and violence is to prevent the episode occurring in the first place. You should discuss the following areas with anyone who asks for your advice:

- avoiding potentially dangerous situations especially when on visits to patients' homes
- learning how to defuse tense confrontations; being able to recognise early warning signs of aggression and being prepared to disarm anger and defuse potentially violent situations
- improving the NHS workplace so that the service provided to patients is efficient, so that patients do not become angry because of long waits or inefficiencies
- devising a workplace policy to handle a violent or aggressive incident
- developing assertiveness and anger management skills
- learning from any violent episode and making changes to avoid a recurrence.

There should be a workplace policy in existence, with which everyone is familiar, to reduce the likelihood of aggression and violence flaring at work, to defuse any such incident effectively, to summon help as necessary, and to counsel and support any victim afterwards.

Activity 5.1: Ask those you appraise to review the safety and security arrangements of their workplace, and plan what they might do if a violent episode does occur. Individuals you appraise (or you, if you are applying this activity to yourself) should circle all the preventive features currently in place in their workplace.[3]

Preventive	**In response to a violent episode**
Staff training	Support staff
Team approach	Report incident
Adequate staffing	Analyse event
Secure premises	Discuss what happened
Surgery alarms	Change systems
Good environment	Review policy
Good communication	Prosecute perpetrator of violence
Workplace policy	Review alarms
Planned interventions for different eventualities	
General awareness of danger	
Good organisation	
Culture of concern for staff	

Then consider what are the most dangerous situations for individuals at work and what changes can they make to minimise the chances of aggression and violence arising?

continued opposite

Potentially threatening situations	Intended changes
•	
•	
•	
•	

Patient safety[4]

As an appraiser you should be aware of the seven steps to patient safety as should anyone working in the NHS. These are:

1 build a safety culture
2 lead and support staff in patient safety matters
3 integrate risk management activity; develop systems and processes to manage risks and identify and assess things that could go wrong
4 promote reporting of incidents
5 involve and communicate with patients and the public
6 learn and share safety lessons
7 implement solutions to prevent harm, through changes to practice, processes or systems.

Your discussions with those you are appraising will be likely to reinforce all aspects of this safety culture.

Ground rules

Look back at Chapter 3 and the section on ground rules. Undertake Activity 3.1 if you did not do that previously or try out the exercise with others you appraise in the future, as appropriate.

Dimension 4. Service development: contribute to development of services (i.e. services for patients and the appraisal process) (Level 3)

Contribute to the development of services to patients through the appraisal process by:

- encouraging reflective practice to enable those you are appraising to learn from their own experiences
- helping others to identify their priorities for service development
- encouraging others being appraised to make improvements to services
- alerting others to the contribution that appraisal and other learning and development can make to the development of services and the NHS. Promote and strengthen the appraisal process
- ensuring that legislation, policies and procedures are applied correctly with regard to appraisal: aware of legal/ethical issues, aware of medico-legal implications.

Consider the extent to which you:

- have the knowledge and skills
- practise them – in your relationship with those you appraise and in your everyday working life in other aspects of your job (you might generalise to 'colleague or member of staff' in the list above).

Complete your audit checklist below in Table 5.2.

Table 5.2: Self-check of own knowledge and skills in respect of service development in relation to appraisal

Aspect of service development	How expert are you? Aware? Competent? Expert?	How frequently do you use these? At least every day? Weekly? Monthly?
Encourage others in reflective practice		
Help others identify priorities for service development		
Encourage individuals to improve services		
Promote and strengthen appraisal process		
Ensure that policies and procedures are applied correctly in relation to appraisal		

How expert are you? Think how expert you are for each aspect of effective service development in relation to appraisal listed in the left-hand column in Table 5.2.

- Aware? If you are merely 'aware' you might be aware that the particular knowledge and/or skill is important and have undertaken some preliminary reading and learning, but are not yet confident, practised or skilled in employing that feature of effective service development.
- Competent? If you are 'competent' you will have a good basic knowledge and be skilled in service development in relation to appraisal.
- Expert? If you are an 'expert' you will have an enormous range of experience and intuitive grasp of situations. You will be able to interpret and synthesise information and handle a wide range of appraisals in different contexts.[2]

How frequently do you use that aspect to achieve effective service development in relation to appraisal? Think how often you employ that feature of effective development with others at work. Is it at least daily or at least weekly or at least monthly? The more such knowledge and skills are part of your normal behaviour, the more likely they will feature naturally and consistently when you meet up with others for their appraisal.

  Make your assessment more objective: seek others' views of your competence or performance. You might simply ask someone else who knows you well to complete the audit Table 5.2 and compare your pre-completed table with their perspective of you – and, of course, discuss any differences with them so that you can learn from their input. You might seek feedback from people whom you appraise or others for whom you have a role or responsibility, such as in line management, educational supervision, mentoring or coaching, or if you are the local lead for the appraisal process.

Reflective practice

Knowles has defined seven fundamentals as guidelines to encourage adult learners in reflective practice, which are relevant to those being appraised.[5]

1 Establish an effective learning climate where people feel safe and comfortable expressing themselves.
2 Involve individuals in mutual planning of relevant methods and curricular content.
3 Trigger internal motivation by involving individuals in diagnosing their own needs.
4 Give others more control by encouraging them to formulate their own learning objectives.
5 Encourage those you are appraising to identify resources and devise strategies for using the resources to achieve their objectives.
6 Support others in carrying out their learning plans.
7 Develop individuals' skills of critical reflection by involving them in evaluating their own learning.

Learning should be a continuous process of investigation, exploration, action, reflection and further action.

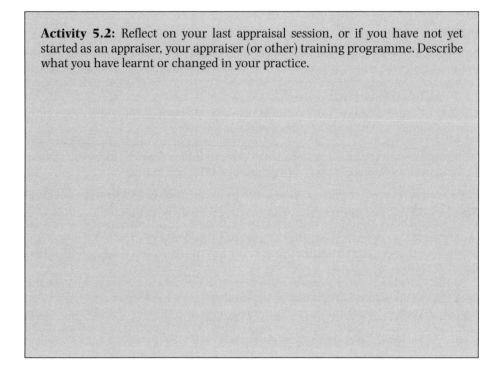

Activity 5.2: Reflect on your last appraisal session, or if you have not yet started as an appraiser, your appraiser (or other) training programme. Describe what you have learnt or changed in your practice.

Strengths, Weaknesses, Opportunities and Threats (SWOT) analysis during the appraisal: help others to identify priorities for service development and improve services

This classic strategic planning technique can be used by you or those you appraise to analyse your or their internal capability, and to set that in relation to service development in relation to work.

Undertake a SWOT analysis of your own performance or that of your team or employing organisation, or encourage those you are appraising to do the same. Work the SWOT analysis up on your own, or with those you are appraising, or with a group of colleagues. Brainstorm the strengths, weaknesses (or challenges), opportunities and threats of your situation.

Strengths and weaknesses of individuals might include: knowledge, experience, expertise, decision making, communication, inter-professional relationships, political skills, timekeeping, organisation, teaching and research. Strengths and weaknesses for the organisation might relate to most of these aspects too, as well as resources – staff, skills or structural items.

Opportunities might relate to unexploited potential strengths, expected changes, options for career development pathways, hobbies and interests that could usefully be expanded.

Threats will include factors and circumstances that prevent you or others from achieving your/their aims for personal, professional and team development, and improvements in patient care.

The SWOT analysis, as with so many of the other learning needs assessment exercises, creates opportunities to learn at the same time as undertaking the actual needs analysis.

Activity 5.3: The person undertaking the SWOT analysis should write on a single flip chart/sheet of paper so that they can see all four quadrants at once.

Strengths	Weaknesses
Opportunities	Threats

Each section is then completed. For example:

1   Strengths – what am I good at? What factors are in my favour?
2   Weaknesses – what am I not so good at?
3   Opportunities – what's likely to be useful that I could harness? What is happening that could help me? What is new, and is it good for me?
4   Threats – what could be a threat to my/our achievements? What's new and is it bad for me?

Prioritise important factors. Draw up goals and a timed action plan.

Now compare what you produced, if working on your own, with what a colleague thought when they addressed the same task. Discuss any differences with them. Describe what you need to learn more about to address the goals you have set for improvement of your knowledge, skills or service provision in relation to the topic(s) you have been considering.

By the end of the SWOT analysis you or your colleague whom you are appraising should be at the stage where you can move on to consider the following.

• How can you optimise and extend the strengths identified?
• How can you minimise or overcome the weaknesses?
• How can you make most use of the opportunities?
• How can you avoid the threats or counter their effects?

Promoting the impact of appraisal

Use all opportunities to let others know about the local appraisal system and the potential benefits to the individual, appraisers, the organisation responsible for the scheme and the NHS as a whole. Encourage others to consider becoming appraisers if that is appropriate. Complete and return any evaluation forms on time. Contribute to any evaluation report of the appraisal scheme's activities (*see* Chapter 8). Collect information about any difficulties that obstruct the appraisal process or prevent the effectiveness of the appraisal sessions or those you are appraising making the most of subsequent developmental opportunities. Feed these back to the appraisal lead and suggest ways that the difficulties can be overcome. Join any steering group overseeing the appraisal system if you can and help to influence its direction and promotion.

Dimension 5. Quality improvement: demonstrate personal commitment to quality improvement, offering others advice and support as an integral part of appraisal process (Level 4)

Contribute to improving the quality of your and others' work by:

• demonstrating personal commitment to quality improvement
• offering advice and support in relation to quality improvement
• understanding national and local healthcare priorities and how these are relevant to others' circumstances
• monitoring your own quality as an appraiser and taking action to improve your performance in this role.

Consider the extent to which you:

• have the knowledge and skills
• practise them – in your relationship with those you appraise and in your everyday working life in other aspects of your job (you might generalise to 'colleague or member of staff' in the list above).

Complete your audit checklist in Table 5.3.

   How expert are you? Think how expert you are for each aspect of quality improvement in relation to appraisal listed in the left-hand column of Table 5.3.

• Aware? If you are merely 'aware' you might be aware that the particular knowledge and/or skill is important and have undertaken some preliminary reading and learning, but are not yet confident, practised or skilled in employing that feature of quality improvement.
• Competent? If you are 'competent' you will have a good basic knowledge and be skilled in quality improvement in relation to appraisal.
• Expert? If you are an 'expert' you will have an enormous range of experience and intuitive grasp of situations. You will be able to interpret and synthesise information and tackle a wide range of types of quality improvement in relation to appraisal in different contexts.[2]

Table 5.3: Self-check of own knowledge and skills in respect of quality improvement in relation to appraisal

Aspect of service development	How expert are you? Aware? Competent? Expert?	How frequently do you use these? At least every day? Weekly? Monthly?
Demonstrate your personal commitment to quality improvement		
Offer individuals advice and support in relation to quality improvement		
Understand national and local healthcare priorities and their relevance to others		
Monitor own quality of work as an appraiser and improve your performance		

How frequently do you use that aspect to achieve quality improvement in relation to appraisal? Think how often you employ that feature of effective improvement with others at work. Is it at least daily or at least weekly or at least monthly? The more such knowledge and skills are part of your normal behaviour, the more likely they will feature naturally and consistently when you meet up with others for appraisals.

   Make your assessment more objective: seek others' views of your competence or performance. You might simply ask someone else who knows you well to complete the audit Table 5.3 and compare your pre-completed table with their perspective of you – and, of course, discuss any differences with them so that you can learn from their input. You might seek feedback from individuals you are appraising or others for whom you have a role or responsibility, such as in line management, educational supervision, mentoring or coaching, or as the local appraisal lead.

Quality improvement[6]

Box 5.1 illustrates Deming's 14 points[7] that are crucial to quality improvement. The focus is to engender quality in service provision by valuing the contributions of individuals and teams. Link the taking of responsibility for learning to do things better directly to service improvement and increased patient or user satisfaction.

   You might refer to Deming's points in justifying how you approach quality improvement in your own appraisal portfolio or to help those you appraise to increase their understanding of quality.

Box 5.1: Quality improvement in a learning organisation: Deming's 14 points[7]

Deming's 14 points
1 Create constancy of purpose
2 Adopt the new philosophy
3 Cease dependence on inspection
4 Cease awarding business on price alone
5 Improve continuously and forever
6 Institute training and retraining on the job
7 Adopt and institute leadership
8 Drive out fear
9 Breakdown barriers between staff
10 Eliminate slogans and targets from the workforce
11 Eliminate numerical quotas and goals
12 Remove barriers that rob people of pride in their work
13 Institute a vigorous programme of education and self-improvement
14 Put everyone in the organisation to work on the transformation

---

Organising 360° feedback[8]

As an appraiser you might recommend 360° appraisal to other individuals as a multisource feedback tool that can provide them with information from others on their performance, from their peer group, managers, staff members, working partners and patients. The tool collects together perceptions from a number of different participants, as in Figure 5.1.

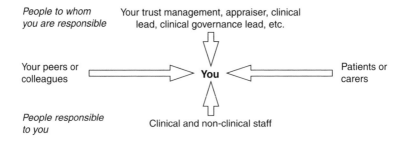

Figure 5.1:   360° feedback.

The wider the spread of people giving feedback, the more rounded the picture. Each individual gives a feedback questionnaire to at least three people included in Figure 5.1. An independent person then collects and collates the questionnaires and discusses the results with the individual. The main disadvantage of this method is that it can sometimes be spoilt by malicious comments against which individuals cannot readily defend themselves.

The NHS Modernisation Agency's Leadership Centre provides a model for a 360° assessment process. For further information about the tool and how to access it go to the website: www.nhsleadershipqualities.nhs.uk/assessment.asp

Significant event analysis[8]

Significant event audit is a structured approach to reviewing events that have occurred at work or in your practice, and was covered in Chapter 2 (*see* page 20). Such events might be in any area of work: prevention, acute care, chronic disease, organisation or management. If a group of colleagues and staff review events together, this allows shared analysis of the issues contributing to the significant event and enables a decision to be made on the implementation of any necessary changes.

Activity 2.5 on page 30 encourages those being appraised to undertake an analysis of a significant event audit.

Dimension 6. Equality, diversity and rights: enable others to exercise their rights and promote equal opportunities and diversity through appraisal (Level 4)

Contribute to the promotion of people's equality, diversity and rights by:

- understanding the principles of equal opportunity and demonstrating best practice in this area
- being aware of your *own* values, beliefs and attitudes and seeking to use these in a constructive manner in the interests of those being appraised
- making evaluations and providing feedback that is free of bias and prejudice; being open and transparent in dealings involving those being appraised
- interpreting people's rights in ways that are consistent with legislation and policies; having a cultural awareness
- demonstrating personal commitment to equality and diversity in respect of your own situation in relating to those you appraise and the service (i.e. staff and patients).

Consider the extent to which you:

- have the knowledge and skills
- practise them – in your relationship with individuals you appraise and in your everyday working life in other aspects of your job (you might generalise to 'colleague or member of staff' in the list above).

Complete your audit checklist in Table 5.4.

How expert are you? Think how expert you are for each aspect of promoting people's equality, diversity and rights in relation to appraisal listed in the left-hand column of Table 5.4.

- Aware? If you are merely 'aware' you might be aware that the particular knowledge and/or skill is important and have undertaken some preliminary reading and learning, but are not yet confident, practised or skilled in employing that feature of promoting people's equality, diversity and rights.
- Competent? If you are 'competent' you will have a good basic knowledge and be skilled in promoting people's equality, diversity and rights in relation to appraisal.

Table 5.4:   Self-check of own knowledge and skills in respect of promoting people's equality, diversity and rights in relation to appraisal and other work settings

Aspect of service development	How expert are you? Aware? Competent? Expert?	How frequently do you use these? At least every day? Weekly? Monthly?
Understand principles of equal opportunity and demonstrate best practice		
Use awareness of *own* values, beliefs and attitudes in constructive manner		
Make evaluations and provide feedback free of bias and prejudice; be open and transparent		
Interpreting rights consistent with legislation and policies; having cultural awareness		
Demonstrating personal commitment to equality and diversity		

- Expert? If you are an 'expert' you will have an enormous range of experience and intuitive grasp of situations. You will be able to interpret and synthesise information and handle promoting people's equality, diversity and rights in different contexts.[2]

How frequently do you promote people's equality, diversity and rights in relation to appraisal and other work settings? Think how often you employ that feature with others at work. Is it at least daily or at least weekly or at least monthly? The more such knowledge and skills are part of your normal behaviour, the more likely they will feature naturally and consistently when you meet up with others in connection with appraisals.

   Make your assessment more objective: seek others' views of your competence or performance. You might simply ask someone else who knows you well to complete the audit Table 5.4 and compare your pre-completed table with their perspective of you – and, of course, discuss any differences with them so that you can learn from their input. You might seek feedback from those you appraise or others for whom you have a role or responsibility, such as in line management, educational supervision, mentoring or coaching, or as the local lead for appraisal.

Equal opportunities

The principle of equal opportunity should apply to employment, training, education, provision of goods, facilities or services. The principle of equal treatment guarantees freedom from discrimination on the grounds of sex, pregnancy, marital status, family status and gender reassignment.[9]

Value diversity – for it is the contrast and differences in views, style, attitudes, ethnic origins, life experiences and personality between people that provides energy and ideas. Exposing elements of diversity can be potentially threatening, as people fear elements of themselves they would rather keep secret may be exposed (look back at the thinking around the façade and blind area in the JoHari window model on page 66). So be sensitive to diversity.

Giving effective feedback

Look back at page 70 to remind yourself of the principles and practice of giving constructive and fair feedback that is free of bias and prejudice.

Being open and transparent

Turn back to page 69 to reflect further on how to establish trust and build open and transparent relationships with those you appraise, or other colleagues.

Activity 5.4

Turn to Chapter 8 and read through the different approaches to evaluation. Pick a method described there and evaluate whether the last person/people you have appraised believe that you (i) gave them constructive feedback, (ii) felt they could trust you with confidences.

Dimension 7. Promotion of self-care and peer support: encourage others to promote their own health and wellbeing through the appraisal process (Level 1)

Contribute to the promotion of the health and wellbeing of others by:

- encouraging individuals whom you appraise to promote their own current and future health and wellbeing
- being sensitive to others' health concerns that may impair their performance and/ or judgement.

Consider the extent to which you:

- have the knowledge and skills
- practise them – in your relationship with those whom you appraise and in your everyday working life in other aspects of your job (you might generalise to 'colleague or member of staff' in the list above).

Complete your audit checklist in Table 5.5.

Table 5.5:   Self-check of own knowledge and skills in promotion of the health and wellbeing of others as part of appraisal

Aspect of service development	How expert are you? Aware? Competent? Expert?	How frequently do you use these? At least every day? Weekly? Monthly?
Encourage others to promote their own current and future health and wellbeing		
Be sensitive to others' health problems that may impair performance and/or judgement		

How expert are you? Think how expert you are in promoting the health and wellbeing of others as listed in the left-hand column of Table 5.5.

- Aware? If you are merely 'aware', you might be aware that the particular knowledge and/or skill is important and have undertaken some preliminary reading and learning, but are not yet confident, practised or skilled in promoting the health and wellbeing of others.
- Competent? If you are 'competent' you will have a good basic knowledge and be skilled in promotion of the health and wellbeing of individuals whom you appraise.
- Expert? If you are an 'expert' you will have an enormous range of experience and intuitive grasp of situations. You will be able to interpret and synthesise information, and promote the health and wellbeing of individuals in different contexts and circumstances.[2]

How frequently do you promote the health and wellbeing of others? Think how often you promote the health and wellbeing of those whom you appraise or that of others at work. Is it at least daily or at least weekly or at least monthly? The more such knowledge and skills are part of your normal behaviour, the more likely they will feature naturally and consistently when you meet up with others who are connected with appraisal.

   Make your assessment more objective: seek others' views of your competence or performance. You might simply ask someone else who knows you well to complete the audit Table 5.5. Compare your pre-completed table with their perspective of you – and, of course, discuss any differences with them so that you can learn from their input. You might seek feedback from individuals you have appraised or others for whom you have a role or responsibility, such as in line management, educational supervision, mentoring or coaching, or as the local lead for appraisal.

Promotion of health and wellbeing of those whom you appraise

Read through the various helpful approaches in Chapter 2. These are aimed at those being appraised, and you can reinforce the importance of them making time and focusing energy on looking after themselves and staying healthy. They may welcome the opportunity to seek your objective input on the way they balance their work and home lives, and deal with competing priorities. You should be in a position to signpost them to other sources of help for stress and health problems.

The NHS has much more emphasis on staff wellbeing these days through the Improving Working Lives (IWL) initiatives developing in every trust. So it may be worth your finding out more about how local or national IWL initiatives could help.

Handling health problems that may impair performance or judgement

It is possible, but very unlikely, that from what you hear during appraisal discussions you, as an appraiser, may have serious concerns about the safety of patients cared for by those you are appraising, due to their health problems. Figure 4.4 (*see* page 71) lists some health-related reasons why a professional's competence might be impaired. These include problems with misuse of alcohol or illicit substances, mental health problems such as having psychosis without any insight, and severe depression.

Persuading an impaired individual to see his or her own GP and follow his or her management will probably be the best course of action. Do not get involved yourself in giving health advice or treatment to individuals you are appraising – it is not your responsibility to do so.

If a situation did crop up where you became aware that patient safety was at risk from the impaired individual and they persist in remaining at work, you should know how to act along the lines discussed under 'Maintaining confidentiality' (*see* page 107).

Activity 5.5

Undertake a significant event audit of an incident where you considered patient safety might be at risk.

Dimension 8. Ability to manage the appraisal process: process and manage data and information and maintain confidentiality (Level 3)

Contribute to processing and managing data and information in relation to appraisal by:

- demonstrating good practice in processing data and information
- sending off data and information to the right place, in a timely way and meaningful format
- presenting evidence of others' performance and learning/service development needs
- taking appropriate action when there are problems with managing and processing data and information
- maintaining confidentiality unless required by duty or statute to do otherwise.

Consider the extent to which you:

- have the knowledge and skills
- practise them – in your relationship with the individual you are appraising and in your everyday working life in other aspects of your job (you might generalise to 'colleague or member of staff' in the list above).

Complete your audit checklist in Table 5.6.

Table 5.6: Self-check of own knowledge and skills in processing and managing data in relation to appraisal

Aspect of service development	How expert are you? Aware? Competent? Expert?	How frequently do you use these? At least every day? Weekly? Monthly?
Demonstrating good practice in processing data and information		
Sending data and information in timely and meaningful format		
Presenting evidence of others' performance and development needs		
Taking appropriate action when problems with data and information occur		
Maintaining confidentiality		

How expert are you? Think how expert you are in processing and managing data as listed in the left-hand column of Table 5.6.

- Aware? If you are merely 'aware' you might be aware that the particular knowledge and/or skill is important and have undertaken some preliminary reading

and learning, but are not yet confident, practised or skilled in processing and managing data in relation to appraisal.
* Competent? If you are 'competent' you will have a good basic knowledge and be skilled in processing and managing data in relation to appraisal.
* Expert? If you are an 'expert' you will have an enormous range of experience and intuitive grasp of situations. You will be able to interpret and synthesise information, and process and manage data in different contexts and circumstances relating to appraisal.[2]

How frequently do you process and manage data and information as part of the appraisal process? Think how often you process and manage data and information. Is it at least daily or at least weekly or at least monthly? The more such knowledge and skills are part of your normal activities, the more likely they will feature naturally and consistently when you meet up with others who are connected with appraisal.

Make your assessment more objective: seek others' views of your competence or performance. You might simply ask someone else who knows you well to complete the audit Table 5.6 and compare your pre-completed table with their perspective of you – and, of course, discuss any differences with them so that you can learn from their input. You might seek feedback from those you have appraised or others for whom you have a role or responsibility, such as in line management, educational supervision, mentoring or coaching, or as the local lead for appraisal.

Demonstrating good practice in processing data and information

The document *Good Medical Practice* guides doctors about standards of record keeping which apply just as much to their role as an appraiser as a clinician. The guidance applies just as much to non-doctors too. They must: 'be honest and trustworthy when writing reports, completing or signing forms, or providing evidence in litigation or other formal inquiries'.[10] This means that individuals must take reasonable steps to verify any statement before they sign a document. They must not write or sign documents which are false or misleading because they omit relevant information. If they have agreed to prepare a report, complete or sign a document, or provide evidence, they must do so without unreasonable delay.

As an appraiser, you will probably find it useful to keep notes on the various issues as they are discussed in the appraisal. Then you and the individual being appraised can come to a joint decision about what goes in the action plan. These notes should be confidential to you both, but will inform the individual's personal development plan (PDP) and the written overview of the appraisal.

Activity 5.6

You could ask the clinical governance lead in your PCO to whom you submit your reports of appraisals, or individuals being appraised themselves, to comment on your standards of completeness or accuracy of the appraisal documentation. Review six such commentaries and see if there are trends or common gaps.

Sending off data and information in timely and meaningful format

It is good practice to complete and submit individual reports and anonymised information about staff learning needs arising from appraisals to the primary care organisation (PCO) or trust (PCT) within a certain time, e.g. two weeks after completing the appraisal.

Presenting evidence of others' performance and development needs

An appraiser will review with those they appraise whether they:

- 'keep clear, accurate, legible and contemporaneous patient records which report the relevant clinical findings, the decisions made, the information given to patients and any drugs or other treatment prescribed
- keep colleagues well informed when sharing the care of patients'.[10]

The written overview of an appraisal should include:

- a concise account of what has been achieved in the last year
- the objectives for the action plan for the next year
- the essential elements for their PDP
- any action required by the practice or PCO to meet local needs or those of the wider community.

Both the individual being appraised and you as appraiser should sign to say that you agree that the appraisal has been carried out correctly. Both of you should keep copies of all these documents. In addition, copies of the appraisal summary, signed by both of you, should be sent to the chief executive and to the clinical governance lead or senior clinical lead of your PCO (depending on local arrangements). These documents are *confidential* and *must* be held securely. Access and use must comply with the Data Protection Act.

Activity 5.7

Review the time taken to complete paperwork and submit the required extracts to the PCO after the next consecutive six (for example) appraisals have been undertaken. Do you need to improve on meeting your deadlines with better time management?

Taking appropriate action when there are problems with data and information

If the appraiser is concerned about someone's performance, they should confer with senior colleagues in the PCO about the appropriate action to take and discuss the situation with the medical director, appraisal lead on the professional executive committee (PEC) of the PCO (or equivalent across the UK) or chief executive (depending on local arrangements). It may be appropriate for the professional regulatory body to be notified. There should be local procedures for suspected or proven underperformance, and the appraiser can hand the matter over to those responsible, according to the agreed protocol. Such suspected underperformance is usually managed by correlating information from all relevant sources and investigating the person's practice further. The appraiser should be well aware of their duties of confidentiality to patients and take care not to breach confidentiality or the regulations of the Data Protection Act when preparing evidence about an individual's underperformance.

Nothing in the appraisal process can take precedence over your professional obligation to protect patients. *See* section on confidentiality below for further consideration of this area.

Activity 5.8

Are there processes in your PCO, to enable you as an appraiser to respond to concerns about the performance of individual members of staff or about the appraisal process or outcome of appraisal? Consider whether there are resources to support the education and development needs of those identified as underperforming by the appraisal, and to make the changes required by the service developments identified and agreed in the appraisal.

Maintaining confidentiality

One of the basic ground rules between you and individuals you appraise will be to agree the extent of the confidential nature of the appraisal discussions and appraisal records, and to build trust between you. But there are limits to confidentiality that should be explicit within the ground rules. It would be unusual for serious problems with an individual's performance to become apparent for the first time during an appraisal. But as an appraiser you would be especially worried about someone who is underperforming in some significant way(s) and appears to have no insight into their weaknesses, and no plans to improve.

Professionals working in the NHS must protect patients when they believe that a colleague's health conduct or performance is a threat to patients. This is clearly laid out in the Department of Health and the GMC's joint guidance on appraisal for doctors (*see* www.revalidationuk.info) and is generalisable to other groups of staff. Therefore, if as a result of an appraisal you believe that the activities of the individual being appraised are such as to put patients at risk, the appraisal process should be stopped and appropriate action taken.

Such action will depend on the person's post and responsibilities, but may include informing and providing evidence to his or her professional body, or a senior person in his or her employing organisation. There is nothing that can override your basic professional obligation to protect patients. You may wish to discuss your problem with the lead for appraisal if you are puzzled as to what action to take.

Dimension 9. Ability to carry out needs assessment: interpret, analyse and synthesise data and information appropriately, within appraisal process (Level 3)

Contribute to producing and communicating information and knowledge by:

- interpreting and synthesising data and information appropriately for appraiser role, recognising limitations of data provided by those being appraised
- being able to distinguish between 'excellent', 'good enough' and 'unacceptable' standards of information and evidence in an appraisal portfolio
- being able to recognise and acknowledge where learning has occurred since the previous appraisal and whether it has addressed the individual's needs
- checking others' understanding of their data included in their individual appraisal portfolios, and its strengths and flaws.

Consider the extent to which you:

- have the knowledge and skills
- practise them – in your relationship with those you appraise and in your everyday working life in other aspects of your job (you might generalise to 'colleague or member of staff' in the list above).

Complete your audit checklist in Table 5.7.

Table 5.7: Self-check of own knowledge and skills in producing and communicating information and knowledge

Aspect of service development	How expert are you? Aware? Competent? Expert?	How frequently do you use these? At least every day? Weekly? Monthly?
Interpreting and synthesising data and information		
Being able to distinguish between 'excellent', 'good enough' and 'unacceptable' standards		
Being able to recognise where learning has occurred since previous appraisal and whether it addressed individual's needs		
Checking others' understanding of data provided for appraisal, its strengths and flaws		

How expert are you? Think how expert you are in producing and communicating information and knowledge in respect of appraisal as listed in the left-hand column of Table 5.7.

- Aware? If you are merely 'aware' you might be aware that the particular knowledge and/or skill is important and have undertaken some preliminary reading and learning, but are not yet confident, practised or skilled in producing and communicating information and knowledge.
- Competent? If you are 'competent' you will have a good basic knowledge and be skilled in producing and communicating information and knowledge.
- Expert? If you are an 'expert' you will have an enormous range of experience and intuitive grasp of situations. You will be able to interpret and synthesise information in different contexts and circumstances.[2]

How frequently do you produce and communicate information and knowledge? Think how often you produce and communicate information and knowledge in relation to appraisal. Is it at least daily or at least weekly or at least monthly with your colleagues or others at work? The more such knowledge and skills are part of your normal behaviour, the more likely they will feature naturally and consistently when you meet up with others who are connected with appraisal.

   Make your assessment more objective: seek others' views of your competence or performance. You might simply ask someone else who knows you well to complete the audit Table 5.7 and compare your pre-completed table with their perspective of you – and, of course, discuss any differences with them so that you can learn from their input. You might seek feedback from those you appraise or others for whom you have a role or responsibility, such as in line management, educational supervision, mentoring or coaching, or as the local lead for appraisal.

Interpreting and synthesising data and information

Data and information you glean from your discussion with the individual being appraised and their documentation is only one piece of information, one snapshot of performance, focusing on a small part of his or her world. The information has to be taken in context and judged for its relevance to the wider work.

Distinguishing between 'excellent', 'good enough' and 'unacceptable' standards

The definition of 'excellent' in the publication *Good Medical Practice for General Practitioners* is being 'consistently good'.[11] This might be a suitable approach for an appraiser to consider adopting when reviewing and discussing someone's performance. Underperformance can cover a range of issues such as knowledge, skills, behaviour and attitudes. It is about achieving less than expectations, or performing below the required levels. Underperformance can be defined in terms of accepted local, professional or national standards, i.e. when performance fails to meet explicit required standards. It can also be defined in terms of relative performance, where the performance of the individual concerned is that of an outlier when compared with that of his or her peers. A single incident will not normally constitute underperformance but repeated less important infringements may. *Good Medical Practice for GPs* describes *unacceptable* practice of clinicians across all areas of work. Some examples are that the *unacceptable* clinician:

- provides better care to some patients than others as a result of his or her own prejudices
- does not acknowledge or attempt to rectify any mistakes that occur
- does not know what skills team members have
- does not refer patients when specialist care is necessary.

The appraiser may detect unacceptable practice from the audits within someone's appraisal portfolio, or from other data collated by the PCO, for example.

Recognising where learning has occurred since previous appraisal and whether learning has addressed someone's needs – as part of appraisal discussion

Look back at Box 3.1 to remind yourself of the way you might structure questions about your colleague's progress since the previous appraisal. Ask them to pick out the most personally significant experiences and what they learned from their experiences. This will involve reflecting on their working lives since their previous appraisal and considering:

- what was most significant
- why this was personally significant
- what they learned from their experiences, reflections or educational events
- any actions they took as a result.

Discuss the extent to which the individual being appraised has applied their learning in making improvements and changes to their own practice, or improved service development in general.

Checking others' understanding of data in appraisal portfolio, its strengths and flaws

As an appraiser, you should be able to help those you appraise realise the extent of their achievements and boost their job satisfaction so that they take professional pride in their work. But you should also be able to help them recognise if they are under-performing and find solutions – which will depend on the reason for the under-performance. In discussing flaws in performance indicated by data collected by those being appraised or the PCO, explore areas that are:

- specific to the individual concerned
- related to the area of concern
- measurable (with agreed methods of measurement)
- based on agreed indicators
- clear, simple and understood
- within well-defined timescales.

The range of interventions might include:

- providing support through peer discussions, suggesting mentoring, etc.
- re-assessment of training and development needs and programmes to meet those needs
- agreeing short-term action plans with performance targets
- a programme to build self-esteem and assertiveness
- training programmes to change attitudes
- changing the environment to suit the needs of the individual
- formal disciplinary measures used as a last resort or reserved for serious cases.

Dimension 10. Ability to contribute to and/or co-ordinate the support system for the appraisal process: develop and sustain partnership working with those appraised and the practice/PCO/Deanery (as appropriate) (appraiser Level 2; appraiser lead Level 4)

Contribute to participating in partnership working in relation to appraisal by:

- developing and sustaining partnership working between appraiser, those being appraised and the organisation
- fostering teamwork and good working relationships with other parts of the health service.

Consider the extent to which you:

- have the knowledge and skills
- practise them – in your relationship with those you appraise and in your everyday working life in other aspects of your job (you might generalise to 'colleague or member of staff' in the list above).

Complete your audit checklist in Table 5.8.

Table 5.8:   Self-check of own knowledge and skills in respect of participation in partnership working in relation to appraisal

Aspect of service development	How expert are you? Aware? Competent? Expert?	How frequently do you use these? At least every day? Weekly? Monthly?
Develop and sustain partnership working between appraiser, those appraised and employing practice or organisation		
Foster teamwork and good working relationships with other parts of NHS		

How expert are you? Think how expert you are for each aspect of participation in partnership working in relation to appraisal listed in the left-hand column of Table 5.8.

*   Aware? If you are merely 'aware' you might be aware that the particular knowledge and/or skill is important and have undertaken some preliminary reading and learning, but are not yet confident, practised or skilled in participating in partnership working in relation to appraisal.
*   Competent? If you are 'competent' you will have a good basic knowledge and be skilled in participating in partnership working in relation to appraisal.
*   Expert? If you are an 'expert' you will have an enormous range of experience and intuitive grasp of situations. You will be able to interpret and synthesise information and participate in partnership working in relation to appraisal in different contexts.[2]

How frequently do you participate in partnership working in relation to appraisal? Think how often you employ partnership working with others at work. Is it at least daily or at least weekly or at least monthly? The more such knowledge and skills are part of your normal behaviour, the more likely they will feature naturally and consistently when you meet up with others who are connected with appraisal.

Make your assessment more objective: seek others' views of your competence or performance. You might simply ask someone else who knows you well to complete the audit Table 5.8 and compare your pre-completed table with their perspective of you – and, of course, discuss any differences with them so that you can learn from their input. You might seek feedback from those you have appraised or others for whom you have a role or responsibility, such as in line management, educational supervision, mentoring or coaching, or as the local lead for appraisal.

Working in teams[12]

You should focus on encouraging common understanding of people's roles, responsibilities and capabilities in helping others understand the benefits of teamworking and working in partnership.

One way to help people understand more about how they perform in a certain role within a team is to use psychometric or psychological measurements or an interpersonal assessment such as the Belbin self-perception inventory.[13] Although teams are made up of individuals, each member fulfils a different role. Different situations dictate the role an individual will adopt and in some situations roles may be duplicated, or one person will play a combination of roles. All roles will be in evidence in any effective social or work group, although it is possible for groups to survive and achieve some of their objectives with one or more of the roles unfilled.

The eight roles identified by Belbin in a 'winning team' are:

*   chairman or co-ordinator: co-ordinating leadership, clarifies goals and priorities
*   plant: generator of ideas, solves difficult problems
*   monitor or evaluator: 'sifter' of ideas, sees all options, analyses, judges likely outcomes
*   team worker: looks after internal relationships, listens, handles difficult people
*   resource investigator: looks after the external relationships, networking, explores new possibilities
*   company worker: loyal to the group, organises, turns ideas and plans into practical forms of action

- shaper: challenges, pressurises, finds ways round obstacles
- completer finisher: ensures tasks and projects are completed, keeps others to schedules and targets.

Activity 5.9

You might encourage those whom you appraise to complete the Belbin inventory and find out more about the role(s) they prefer to play in a team, if that is relevant.

Working in partnerships

People are more likely to learn about the benefits of working in partnerships and develop new meaningful partnerships themselves by observing others as successful role models. Listed below are the positive features of partnerships that are most likely to be successful. Good partnerships between staff of different disciplines or the NHS and other organisations, such as those in the voluntary sector or social services, depend on creating trust, mutual respect and joint working for common goals:[12]

- a written memorandum of partnership
- a joint strategy with agreed goals and outcomes
- widespread support by individuals working within the partnership and their organisations
- clear roles and responsibilities with respect to joint working
- shared decision making on partnership matters
- each partner has different attributes which fit well with the other partner
- the partnership benefits all contributors
- the whole partnership is greater than the sum of the components
- each partner makes a 'fair' investment in the partnership – and the risk/benefit balance between partners is fair
- partners trust each other and are honest over partnership matters
- partners appreciate, respect and tolerate each others' differences
- there is a common understanding about language and communication.

Activity 5.10

Encourage the person you are appraising to shadow someone else who holds a post to which they aspire or would benefit from knowing more about, so that they can get real insights about another job or sector or type of work. Ask them to reflect on how this will influence their career or development plan.

Dimension 11. Leadership skills: lead others in the development of knowledge, ideas and work practice as an integral part of the appraisal process (Level 2)

Contribute to the development of leadership by:

- leading and inspiring those you appraise in the development of their knowledge, ideas and work practice
- recognising your own leadership skills and those of others.

Consider the extent to which you:

- have the knowledge and skills
- practise them – in your relationship with others and in your everyday working life in other aspects of your job (you might generalise to 'colleague or member of staff' in the list above).

Complete your audit checklist in Table 5.9.

Table 5.9: Self-check of own knowledge and skills in respect of leadership in relation to appraisal and everyday work

Aspect of service development	How expert are you? Aware? Competent? Expert?	How frequently do you use these? At least every day? Weekly? Monthly?
Lead and inspire others in development of knowledge, ideas and work practice		
Recognise own leadership skills and those of others		

How expert are you? Think how expert you are for each aspect of the development of leadership in relation to appraisal listed in the left-hand column of Table 5.9.

- Aware? If you are merely 'aware' you might be aware that the particular knowledge and/or skill is important and have undertaken some preliminary reading and learning, but are not yet confident, practised or skilled in developing leadership.
- Competent? If you are 'competent' you will have a good basic knowledge and be skilled in leadership in relation to appraisal.
- Expert? If you are an 'expert' you will have an enormous range of experience and intuitive grasp of situations. You will be able to interpret and synthesise information and provide leadership in relation to appraisal in different contexts.[2]

How frequently do you provide leadership in relation to appraisal or your everyday work? Is it at least daily or at least weekly or at least monthly with your colleagues or others at work? The more such knowledge and skills are part of your normal behaviour, the more likely they will feature naturally and consistently when you meet up with others who are connected with appraisal.

Make your assessment more objective: seek others' views of your competence or performance. You might simply ask someone else who knows you well to complete the audit Table 5.9 and compare your pre-completed table with their perspective of you – and, of course, discuss any differences with them so that you can learn from their input. You might seek feedback from those you have appraised or others for whom you have a role or responsibility, such as in line management, educational supervision, mentoring or coaching, or as the local appraisal lead.

Leadership styles

Leaders include those people in your practice or PCO who have responsibility for developing vision, strategic planning, organisational performance, redesign and extension of services, service quality and workforce development.

One type of leadership is to direct and co-ordinate the work of others to build, support and work with teams, to work effectively as part of a team, and to negotiate and consult effectively. This type of leadership emphasises the 'democratic' concept of team leadership. A team leader with a democratic style enables a team to function well and encourages rather than imposes change.[6]

Leadership styles vary greatly, ranging from authoritarian to developmental (*see* Box 5.2). The categories are not mutually exclusive, and each style is relevant in the appropriate context.

Box 5.2:   Leadership styles[14]

1   **Authoritarian**: giving clear directions for specific tasks
2   **Authoritative**: stating broad objectives and delegating the detailed execution to others while accepting responsibility for the outcome
3   **Democratic**: encouraging participation to secure the benefit of the expertise of all team members
4   **Task-oriented**: focusing on the task in hand and requiring high standards in accomplishment of tasks, regardless of other considerations
5   **Developmental**: focusing on the longer-term development of members of the team as an investment in the future

---

Activity 5.11

Reflect on what type of leader style describes you and why. Discuss your self-analysis at your next appraisal with your line manager or own appraiser and seek their insights and suggestions as to how you might change your leadership style, if that is appropriate.

Leaders in health settings[15-17]

- Develop and articulate a vision. They show how the vision can be realised and engage people in developing the vision and seeing that the vision is reflected in strategies and action.
- Motivate others. They design jobs so that people perform well. They invest time and energy in supporting and listening to people. They know how to motivate people and encourage high standards.
- Make decisions. They seek the views and opinions of key people and engage others in taking decisions. They are prepared to take difficult and unpopular decisions.
- Release others' talents. They identify and overcome barriers for individuals, teams and organisations in achieving their potential.
- Demonstrate responsiveness and flexibility. They are able to react positively and competently to an unexpected event themselves, and develop a culture of flexibility and responsiveness in the organisation as priorities change.
- Embody a set of values. They make the values of the organisation clear to others internally and externally. They work towards equity and access to services and are good role models themselves as regarding their conduct and personal behaviour.
- Innovate. They encourage a culture where creativity and innovation are welcomed and people learn from past successes or failures. They try out new ideas.
- Work across boundaries. They are committed to working in partnership and overcoming barriers to joint working.
- Demonstrate resilience and assistance. They demonstrate self-confidence themselves, and build confidence in individuals and teams.

Activity 5.12: Seek feedback from other colleagues about the nature of your leadership skills and practice. Ask them to make comments about how you perform as a leader against the headings from Box 5.2.

Develop and articulate a vision

Motivate others

Make decisions

Release others' talents

continued opposite

Are responsive and flexible

Embody a set of values

Innovate

Work across boundaries

Are resilient

Build others' confidence

And lastly ... protected time: identify and negotiate protected time to devote to the appraisal process

This twelfth requirement of appraisers is not a dimension within the NHS KSF, but it is a practical requirement for an appraiser to be able to devote sufficient dedicated time to his or her role in appraisal and follow-up reviews.

An appraiser should be able to demonstrate through record keeping and feedback from others that they:

- make time for the individuals whom they appraise and their follow-up action plans
- take an active part in local learning sets, which provide peer support for appraisers and others in connection with appraisal.

References

1   Department of Health (2003) *The NHS Knowledge and Skills Framework (NHS KSF) and Development Review Guidance – Working Draft. Version 6.* Department of Health, London.

2   Benner P (1984) *From Novice to Expert.* Addison-Wesley, London.

3   Chambers R (1998) *Survival Skills for GPs.* Radcliffe Medical Press, Oxford.

4   National Patient Safety Agency (2003) *Seven Steps to Patient Safety. A Guide for NHS Staff.* National Patient Safety Agency, London.

5   Knowles MS (1984) *Andragogy in Action: applying modern principles of adult learning.* Jossey-Bass, San Francisco, CA.

6   Garcarz W, Chambers R and Ellis S (2003) *Make Your Healthcare Organisation a Learning Organisation.* Radcliffe Medical Press, Oxford.

7   Deming WE (1986) *Out of the Crisis.* Cambridge University Press, Cambridge.

8   Chambers R, Wakley G, Field S and Ellis S (2003) *Appraisal for the Apprehensive.* Radcliffe Medical Press, Oxford.

9   Equal Opportunities Commission (1998) *Equality in the 21st Century.* Equal Opportunities Commission, Manchester.

10 General Medical Council (2001) *Good Medical Practice.* GMC, London.

11 Royal College of General Practitioners/General Practitioners Committee (2002) *Good Medical Practice for General Practitioners.* RCGP, London.

12 Mohanna K, Wall D and Chambers R (2004) *Teaching Made Easy. A manual for health professionals* (2e). Radcliffe Medical Press, Oxford.

13 Belbin RM (1981) *Managerial Teams. Why They Succeed or Fail.* Heinemann, Oxford.

14 Rashid A and McAvoy P (2002) Managing to be a successful leader. *GP.* **30 September**: 40–2.

15 Frances D and Woodcock M (1996) *The Unblocked Manager.* Gower, Aldershot.

16 Scott T (2000) Clinicians in management. In: Leadership in health: a UK perspective on clinical leadership – Part 2. *Healthcare Review Online.* **4(2)**: 1–20.

17 Simpson J (2000) Clinical leadership in the UK. In: Leadership in health: a UK perspective on clinical leadership – Part 2. *Healthcare Review Online.* **4(2)**: 20–6.

6

Demonstrating your competence as an appraiser

In the drive to regulate professionals' standards of practice, everyone must collect and retain information that demonstrates their current competence in their work (*see* Box 6.1 for a definition of competence). So, an appraiser should gather evidence that they are competent and staying up-to-date as an appraiser and in other areas of their work.

Box 6.1:

Competence is: 'able to perform the tasks and roles required to the expected standard'.[1]

Five stages in organising your evidence[2]

The stages of the evidence cycle for demonstrating your standards of practice or competence as an appraiser and any necessary improvements you should make are given in Figure 6.1. Although the five stages are shown in sequence, in practice you would expect to move backwards and forwards from stage to stage, because of new information or a modification of your earlier ideas. A critical incident or complaint from an individual whom you have appraised might occur and cause you to reconsider how you conduct appraisals. The arrows in Figure 6.1 show that you might reset your target or aspirations for good practice having undertaken exercises to identify what you need to learn, or determine whether there are deficiencies in the way you conduct appraisals.[2]

Stage 1: Select your aspirations for good practice

These will be to be a consistently good appraiser whichever individual you are appraising.

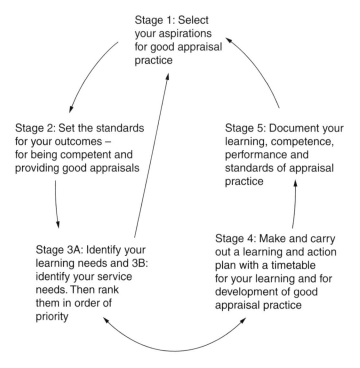

Figure 6.1: Stages of the evidence cycle.

Stage 2: Set the standards of your outcomes, for being competent and providing a good service

Outcomes might include:

- the way that learning is applied (e.g. in applying your knowledge and skills of appraisal)
- a learned skill (*see* Chapters 3 and 4)
- a protocol (e.g. those underpinning the appraisal process in your practice or primary care organisation (PCO); *see* Chapter 9)
- a strategy that is implemented (e.g. the appraisal and learning strategies in your PCO)
- meeting of recommended standards.

You could incorporate into your standards or outcomes those components specified by universities at a national level as part of their Masters Frameworks for their postgraduate awards. The Masters Frameworks consist of eight components that shape the individual postgraduate award programme outcomes and the learning outcomes of the individual modules for the postgraduate awards. The eight components are:

- analysis
- problem solving

- knowledge and understanding
- reflection
- communication
- learning
- application
- enquiry.

You could set out your continuing professional development (CPD) work in the portfolio you are assembling for appraisals in this format. This would help you to document your professional development to date in a form that can be readily 'Accredited for Prior Experiential Learning' (APEL) by universities (contact your local universities if you want more information about this process). You might then be given credits for learning against an intended postgraduate award. It would save you from duplicating work, as well as speeding your progress through the award.

Stage 3: Identify your learning and service needs in your practice or primary care organisation and rank them in order of priority

The type and depth of documentation you need to gather will encompass:

- the context in which you work
- your knowledge and skills in relation to being an appraiser or any other particular role or responsibility that you have.

The extent of expertise you should possess will depend on your level of responsibility for appraisal – are you the appraisal lead in your organisation, do you train other appraisers, do you appraise a variety of people of different seniorities? Your learning needs should take into account your aspirations for the future too – personal or career development for you, or improvements in the way you deliver care in your practice. Refer to Chapter 2 for more ideas on how you will identify your learning or service development needs.

Group and summarise your service development needs from the exercises you have carried out. Grade them according to the priority you set. You may put one at a higher priority because it fits in with service development needs established in the business plan of the trust or practice, or put another lower because it does not fit in with other activities that are included in your organisation's current development plan for the next 12 months. If you have needs identified by several different methods of assessment, then they will have a higher priority than something only identified once.

Look back at your aspirations and standards set out in Stages 1 and 2. Match your learning or service development needs with one or more of these standards, or others that you have set yourself.

Stage 4: Make and carry out a learning and action plan with a timetable for your personal and service development

If you have not identified any learning needs for yourself or the service as a whole, you should omit Stage 4 and tidy up the presentation of your evidence for inclusion in your appraisal portfolio as at the end of Stage 5.

Think about whether:

- you have defined your learning objectives – what you need to learn to be able to attain the standards and outcomes you have described in Stage 2
- you can justify spending time and effort on the topics you prioritised in Stage 3
- you have time and resources for learning about that topic or making the associated changes to service delivery. Check that you are not trying to do too much too quickly, or you will become discouraged
- learning about that topic will make a difference to the way you conduct appraisals or provide care for patients
- you have achieved a good balance across your areas of work or between your personal aspirations and the basic requirements for appraisal or of the service.

Decide on what method of learning is most appropriate for your task or role or the standards you are expecting to attain or sustain. You may have already identified your preferred learning style, but read up on this on page 24 if you are unsure.

Describe how you will carry out your learning plan and what you will do by a specific time. State how your learning will be applied and how and when it will be evaluated. Build in some staging posts so that you do not suddenly get to the end of 12 months and discover that you have only done half of your plan.

Your action plan should also include your role in remedying any gaps in service delivery that you identified in Stage 3 and which are within the remit of your responsibility.

Stage 5: Document your learning, competence, performance and standards of service delivery

You might choose to document that you have attained your defined outcomes by repeating the learning needs assessment that you started with. You could record your increased confidence and competence in dealing with situations that you previously avoided or performed inadequately.

As you start to collate information around this five-stage cycle, discuss any problems about appraisal with colleagues, experts in this area, tutors, etc. You want to develop a wide range and depth of evidence so that you can show that you are competent in your day-to-day general work as well as for your expertise as an appraiser.

There is a difference between being competent and performing in a consistently competent manner. You need to be motivated to perform consistently well and enabled to do so with efficient systems and sufficient resources. You will require sufficient numbers of other staff and available infrastructure for performing well in your day-to-day work, and protected time, good administrative support and training resources to perform well as an appraiser, for example.

The following three examples give illustrative cycles of evidence based on the five-stage cycle, that you might use or adapt to enable you to gather evidence to show that you are performing well as an appraiser. They are reproduced from Chambers *et al.*[2]

Collecting data to demonstrate your learning, competence and performance as an appraiser

Example cycle of evidence

Case Study: Dealing with hostility from someone being appraised

Graham has cancelled his appraisal interview twice at short notice, but you both meet on the third booked date and time. He sent you his completed paperwork one week ago after you had rung to prompt him. What he has sent in is rather sketchy and the personal development plan (PDP) has very little information and does not refer to learning undertaken as a result of last year's version of his PDP. As you start the interview, Graham appears to be hostile and silent.

Stage 1: Select your aspirations for good practice

The excellent appraiser:

- undertakes an honest and fair appraisal.

Stage 2: Set the standards for your outcomes

Outcomes might include:

- the way learning is applied
- a learnt skill
- a protocol
- a strategy that is implemented
- meeting recommended standards.

1 Understand and able to explain the purpose of appraisal and personal development planning.
2 Able to enable others to undertake and maintain a personal development plan.

Stage 3A: Identify own learning needs

1 Informal feedback from Graham at the end of the appraisal and more formal feedback from Graham and others you have appraised, fed back via primary care organisation (PCO).
2 Peer review by doctor or nurse continuing professional development (CPD) tutor about how you explain the purpose and methods of a PDP – captured by trio work, audiocassette taping, etc., with subject's informed consent.
3 Significant event audit in relation to the two cancelled appraisal interview dates.

Stage 3B: Identify your service needs

Any of the needs assessment exercises in Stage 3A may also reveal service needs.

1 Reflections and discussion with other appraisers at appraiser support group run by PCO or Deanery with self-realisation of your own strengths and weaknesses.
2 The remarks in your own feedback from PCO of the doctors appraised compared with other appraisers' feedback.
3 Outcomes of pooling of information from practitioners' PDPs across the trust – looking at themes and patterns that are emerging.

Stage 4: Make and carry out a learning and action plan

1 Attend the ongoing local training and support meetings for appraisers.
2 Attend a local workshop for medical and dental and other healthcare CPD tutors about personal development planning. Run a small group there about best practice.
3 Represent general practice appraisal on the strategic working party of the trust that considers outcomes of PDPs and appraisal and the pooling of information about common themes to inform allocation of resources for education and training activities as well as service developments.
4 Read up on worked examples of PDPs.[4–6]

Stage 5: Document your learning, competence, performance and standards of service delivery

1 Feedback on appraiser performance and your own reflections on that feedback.
2 Record of the peer review conclusions and subsequent action.
3 Minutes of the significant event audit discussion with fellow appraisers and the subsequent action in general, and with Graham in particular.
4 Notes of the strategic working party meetings and action plan.
5 Contents of the workshop on PDPs and flip chart notes emanating from the small group work.

Case Study continued

Graham's initial hostility and fear melted away with your persistent encouragement. He had come expecting to be judged harshly for his lack of evidence of learning or progress in his PDP. When he found you adopted a helpful manner he thawed and the evidence of his learning and striving to improve his performance was teased out. You showed Graham how to compose a PDP in a meaningful way and offered to put him in touch with the local CPD tutor. However, Graham told you that he had already had an offer from one of his colleagues with a 'brilliant' PDP to work alongside her on both PDPs. You arrange to phone him again in two months' time to see how he's getting on.

Example cycle of evidence

> **Case Study:** Being appraised as a teacher
>
> You have been an appraiser for a year, but next month it is your turn to be appraised by a colleague. You check over your portfolio carefully as you want to impress your colleague with how comprehensive and thorough a practitioner you are. You ensure that you include sufficient evidence in your portfolio to show that you are a competent appraiser who performs consistently well, and that you have documented data about your teaching skills in your one-day-a-week post in health informatics at the local university.

Stage 1: Select your aspirations for good practice

The excellent healthcare appraiser and teacher:

- provides information that he or she is a competent appraiser/teacher in a specialty subject
- shows that he or she performs consistently well as an appraiser/teacher in a specialty subject.

Stage 2: Set the standards for your outcomes

Outcomes might include:

- the way learning is applied
- a learnt skill
- a protocol
- a strategy that is implemented
- meeting recommended standards.

1 Good peer review by appraiser of your portfolio who is enthusiastic about your documented work.
2 Evidence of your learners' development in pursuing their health informatics course in relation to teaching by you.

Stage 3A: Identify your learning needs

1 A preview critique of your portfolio by a colleague or 'buddy' when you think it is complete to identify any gaps.
2 Check that all areas are covered within your portfolio: educational, personal and professional development, career progress, key areas of work with both objective and subjective evidence of your competence and performance.
3 Look at the parallel appraisal from the university management of your academic work and reflections on previous appraisal and achievements of last year's development plan for overlaps and gaps.

Stage 3B: Identify your service needs

Any of the needs assessment exercises in Stage 3A may also reveal service needs.

1 The input into the university examining body and personal feedback from the external examiner about the running of the health informatics course.
2 Compare the curriculum taught in health informatics against current NHS requirements for health informatics, looking for gaps or disproportionate emphases in the content of course.

Stage 4: Make and carry out a learning and action plan

1 Attend a local seminar for people preparing for appraisal on how to get the best out of your appraisal, purposely taking the subject's perspective even though you are an appraiser too.
2 Attend an advanced skills course in an aspect of teaching to develop a particular interest or expertise.
3 Plan and undertake educational research into an area of special interest that spans appraisal and teaching activities, e.g. improving interpersonal skills, helping other people to change their behaviour, or enhancing multidisciplinary working.

Stage 5: Document your learning, competence, performance and standards of service delivery

1 Appraisal portfolio and appraiser's report with your agreed action plan.
2 The external examiner's report for the health informatics course, including material relevant to your performance.
3 Appraisal of your performance as a teacher and outstanding training needs from colleague or line manager at university.
4 Certificate of attendance, accreditation or qualifications gained at the teaching skills course.

Case Study continued

You looked forward to your appraisal as the day drew nearer as a chance to talk about your achievements to a colleague who was really interested in all that you had been doing. In the event, it was an even better session than you anticipated as your appraiser posed some challenging questions for you. You ended up talking about where your career was heading, and by the end of the appraisal, when the paperwork was completed, you left with a great deal to think through about your ongoing personal development and potential opportunities.

Example cycle of evidence

Case Study: Separating out poor performance from appraisal

The date of your appraisal with Chris has been fixed for several months, being in the last month of her placement with you. You ask colleagues to complete a 360° feedback questionnaire about Chris, because one or two have hinted that they will be glad to see her move on elsewhere, but you have been too busy until now to ask for any specific information. The only piece of evidence that you have of Chris' poor performance is a recent audit. This revealed that Chris had not acted upon two abnormal results sent back from the laboratory but had simply filed them in the patients' notes.

Soon after the appraisal discussion begins, Chris bursts into tears as she has already seen the 360° feedback report and knows what is coming. However, a brief discussion shows that she lacks insight and feels the staff were wrong to criticise her, and they seem to pick on her unfairly. When challenged about the filing of the abnormal results, Chris declares that it is not attributable to her but the fault of the clerical staff who filed them away. You officially stop the appraisal as Chris is still tearful, but are not sure whether to reconvene another day when Chris has calmed down or if you should be following the poor performance procedures (if you knew what they were).

Stage 1: Select your aspirations for good practice
The excellent appraiser:

- undertakes an honest and fair appraisal
- ensures that patients are not put at risk by practitioners in training.

Stage 2: Set the standards for your outcomes
Outcomes might include:

- the way learning is applied
- a learnt skill
- a protocol
- a strategy that is implemented
- meeting recommended standards.

1   Able to recognise poor performance in a trainee for whom you are responsible at an early stage.
2   Able to minimise or avoid harm to patients or NHS services from poor performance in a trainee or other learner.

Stage 3A: Identify your learning needs
1   Compare audits of the performance of the trainee and colleagues from the same discipline in the workplace.

2 Feedback from colleagues as to your listening skills when they commented on trainee's performance in ad hoc way, e.g. at coffee breaks, when work had been left undone.
3 Read and reflect on methods of formative assessment and whether you know how to, and do, apply those methods to help the trainee understand what performance is expected.

Stage 3B: Identify your service needs

Any of the needs assessment exercises in Stage 3A may also reveal service needs.

1 Phone the lead in the trust or local professional committee about procedures in place for addressing poor performance of clinicians or lead at local training institution where trainee is registered. Read through the current guidance and the steps you should take.
2 Obtain copies of past reports of the trainee's performance, or if this is not possible, discuss your concerns with the previous trainer or person responsible for the trainee's qualifying programme.

Stage 4: Make and carry out a learning and action plan

1 Identifying your personal learning needs or service needs will have provided learning material.
2 Read up about the poor performance procedures in other healthcare organisations – search their websites and that of the General Medical Council or other regulatory bodies.
3 Talk to other trainers to find out if they have had similar problems in the past and how they have confronted poor performance in a trainee with positive outcomes.

Stage 5: Document your learning, competence, performance and standards of service delivery

1 You obtain documentation about the poor performance procedures that exist in your trust with an objective report about Chris and the stages you have embarked upon, the referrals made, the measures taken and the help planned.
2 List of useful websites.
3 Confidential account of Chris' poor performance and notes of discussion with anyone to whom you have referred the case.

Case Study continued

Chris did apologise the next day and explained that she has been distracted at work because of personal problems at home, which she realised she must sort out after the tearful session of the previous day. You arranged to discuss the 360° feedback and inappropriate response to abnormal results at an extra-ordinary tutorial the following week, but still carried on with your cycle of learning about poor performance procedures so that you could be prepared to address Chris' continuing poor performance if necessary.

References

1 Eraut M and du Boulay B (2000) *Developing the Attributes of Medical Professional Judgement and Competence.* University of Sussex, Sussex. Reproduced at www.informatics.sussex.ac.uk/users/bend/doh

2 Chambers R, Mohanna K, Wakley G and Wall D (2004) *Demonstrating Your Competence 1: healthcare teaching.* Radcliffe Medical Press, Oxford.

3 General Medical Council (2001) *Good Medical Practice.* General Medical Council, London.

4 Wakley G, Chambers R and Field S (2000) *Continuing Professional Development in Primary Care: making it happen.* Radcliffe Medical Press, Oxford.

5 Chambers R, Stead J and Wakley G (2001) *Diabetes Matters in Primary Care.* Radcliffe Medical Press, Oxford.

6 Wakley G, Chambers R and Iqbal Z (2001) *Cardiovascular Disease Matters in Primary Care.* Radcliffe Medical Press, Oxford.

7

Linking appraisal with career planning, career development and career enhancement[1]

Career planning is a must at all stages of a health service career; for students or young professionals uncertain of their career paths, for established health professionals and managers faced with a range of career opportunities and dilemmas, or when thinking of retirement. It is likely that career planning and development will be discussed during most appraisals. An appraiser may reflect on his or her career development, too – you may well have become an appraiser as a form of career development if the appraiser role is not a compulsory part of line management.

This chapter presents a basis for you (or those you appraise) to review where you are with your career and plan further developments as appropriate. Alternatively, you might want to guide those you appraise towards career planning or career development.

Your career review

Consider the questions posed below and the items in Box 7.1.

*   Who are you and where are you now?
*   How satisfied are you with your career and life?
*   Are you ready to make a change?

Then plan:

*   where you want to be
*   how you are going to get there
*   what you will do if you do not get there.

Box 7.1: Career life planning

*   Identify relevant experience, personal resources and skills
*   Clarify hopes and ambitions for development
*   Describe potential barriers to achievement
*   Identify career options

Your career plans may centre on developing your particular skills and interests within the discipline and/or specialty in which you are working so that you function more effectively. You may want to develop your career so that you become more specialised in a particular clinical or managerial area. You might want more variety in your work and decide to develop a parallel area of interest or a new skill that enhances your current post. It may be promotion that you are after, with more status or responsibility. You may crave for a complete change in a new career that is a natural extension of your current work, or as a fresh start in a different career within or outside the NHS.

You may be able to self-assess your satisfaction with your career and plan your development, or you may need help in finding out about the career possibilities, or in selecting a career path that will suit you and match your strengths and values. Box 7.2 describes the various sources of help with career development that may be available in your locality.

Box 7.2:   Sources of help with career development[1]

- *Careers information* covers the facts about the qualifications and experience needed for alternative career pathways, and the opportunities that there are for career progression; that is, the number and type of posts available at a particular level and in a particular specialty, and details of the qualifications and training necessary.
- *Careers guidance* is personal and directive, and provides *advice* within the context of the opportunities that are available.
- *Career counselling* is an umbrella term for the process of enabling somebody to evaluate their current situation and identify what steps are needed in order to change. It will usually include identification of a person's strengths and weaknesses in relation to work options, and may also include careers information.
- *Coach, mentor* (*see* page 50).

Factors to consider in *reviewing* or *choosing* a career specialty or interest[2,3]

When reviewing your current job or weighing up the potential for a career move, you should consider the match between you and the job as to whether:

- you have the sort of personality that fits with the requirements of the job
- you have the appropriate skills, training and experience
- you have sufficient job satisfaction and interest in your work
- you are sufficiently motivated to work effectively
- the job fits with your ethics, inner values and boundaries
- the job provides the balance you want between work and your off-duty life.

Reflect on what you are looking for from your work:

- the kind of work you enjoy – routine, exciting, prestigious, quiet and steady
- the setting in which you want to work – community, hospital, rural, urban, travel
- the type of people for whom you want to care – the ages and characteristics of patients

- the type of people with whom you want to work – and whether in a small team or big organisation
- the extent of patient contact that suits you
- the level of income you consider (i) essential and (ii) desirable
- the working hours, holidays, study leave: how the hours fit with your current state and future domestic plans
- opportunities for parallel career interests, such as research, writing, education, consultancy, private work or work-related hobbies
- the extent of professional autonomy and responsibility you want.

You will also need to take account of:

- the details of any training required – hours, practical difficulties, examinations
- the job prospects of alternative career paths: the opportunities for you to progress.

Do not forget the impact of your career choice upon those at home – if that is relevant to your circumstances. Your family may not be tolerant of you prioritising your career, or studying for further qualifications or making a house move to take up a different post.[4]

Job evaluation[5]

The NHS has introduced a job evaluation scheme to help ensure that employed staff are rewarded fairly as part of the Agenda for Change initiative; and ensure that the NHS respects the principles of equal pay for work of equal value.[6] A number of national job profiles have been agreed with specific roles and responsibilities. The factors on which jobs have been evaluated include the following.

1 Communication and relationship skills – where the highest level concerns 'providing and receiving highly complex, sensitive or contentious information where there are significant barriers to acceptance which need to be overcome using the highest level of interpersonal and communication skills'.
2 Knowledge, training and experience – where the highest level involves 'advanced theoretical and practical knowledge of a range of work procedures and practices' or 'specialist knowledge over more than one discipline/function acquired over a significant period'.
3 Analytical and judgemental skills – where the highest level consists of 'judgements involving highly complex facts or situations, which require the analysis, interpretation and comparison of a range of options'.
4 Planning and organisational skills – where the highest level concerns 'formulating long-term, strategic plans which involve uncertainty and which may impact across the whole organisation'.
5 Physical skills – where the highest level requires 'physical skills where a high degree of precision or speed and the highest levels of hand, eye and sensory co-ordination are essential'.
6 Responsibilities for patient/client care – where the highest level is 'corporate responsibility for the provision of a clinical, clinical technical or social care service(s)'.
7 Responsibilities for policy and service development implementation – where the highest level demands 'corporate responsibility for major policy implementation and policy or service development, which impacts across or beyond the organisation'.

8   Responsibilities for financial and physical resources – where the highest level is of 'corporate responsibility for the financial resources and physical assets of an organisation'.

9   Responsibilities for human resources – where the highest level involves 'corporate responsibility for the human resources or HR function'.

10   Responsibilities for information resources.

11   Responsibilities for research and development.

12   Freedom to act – where the highest level involves the interpretation of 'overall health service policy and strategy, in order to establish goals and standards'.

13   Physical effort.

14   Mental effort – where the highest level requires 'intense concentration'.

15   Emotional effort – rating frequency and intensity of exposure to distressing or traumatic circumstances.

16   Working conditions – rating exposure to unpleasant working conditions or hazards.

Describing and rating jobs using these factors enables a much clearer definition of the roles and responsibilities of a post – job titles may be misleading. The Knowledge and Skills Framework (developed for appraisers in Chapters 4 and 5) underpins the job evaluation scheme.[7]

Job satisfaction and career fulfilment

Job satisfaction is known to protect health professionals from the effects of stress from work, so increasing your job satisfaction is one of the best ways to 'stress-proof' yourself against the pressures and demands of a job. You will minimise the effects of the elements of the job you find more stressful if you enjoy your job, feel valued and are in control of your everyday work. Low job satisfaction can affect your performance.[2]

Appreciating your personal ethics and work values

Your ethics set the boundaries as to how far you are prepared to go to get what you want. Work values are personal to you too. You will be happiest and most fulfilled in a job that incorporates your main work values. Eight career anchor categories have been identified by Schein[8] to increase people's insights into their strengths and motivation as part of career development. These are:

- technical or functional competence
- general managerial competence
- autonomy or independence
- security or stability
- entrepreneurial creativity
- service or dedication to a cause
- pure challenge
- lifestyle.

People define their self-image in terms of these traits and come to understand more about their talents, motives and values – and which of these they would not give up if forced to make a choice.

Motivation

People are motivated by different things. Money, fame and power are all key motivators. Pride, lust, anger, gluttony, envy, sloth and covetousness are all listed as prime motivators – hopefully not all of these are relevant to any great extent in the NHS! Some of the best motivators for fulfilling health professionals' and managers' needs are:

- interesting and/or useful work
- sense of achievement
- responsibility
- opportunities for career progression or professional development
- gaining new skills or competencies
- sense of belonging to a primary care unit or practice team or the NHS.

We know that self-esteem and fulfilment are not possible if the basic structure and safety components of your life are not secure. Self-esteem, status and recognition from others are only possible if they are built on a good social base that includes love, friendship, belonging to groups (work, home, leisure, professional) and social activities. Fulfilment, maturity and wisdom are only possible where all the other conditions encourage growth, personal development and accomplishment.

Relationship between continuing professional development and career development

Career development should be an integral part of your personal development plan (PDP), setting out goals for the forthcoming year and beyond, and realistic ways of achieving those goals. An annual appraisal or a performance review is a good time to review your plan – by your appraiser, a trusted colleague, a mentor or line manager.

You cannot consider your own individual needs and plans in isolation from those of the rest of your work team or organisation, or the needs of the NHS as a whole. There needs to be an opening for such a post or the new skills you intend to develop. A successful PDP must balance competing influences and pressures of service needs and NHS priorities while enabling individual practitioners to *stay in control* of the development of their careers and working lives, and retain their organisation's and colleagues' support.

Activity 7.1: Where are you now? Career review and assessment[1]

You might do this analysis of your skills and strengths, plans and vision by yourself or with a mentor, tutor or trusted colleague. You might use the exercises to help someone else.

Looking inwards

You
- What are your strengths and weaknesses as a health professional or manager?
- Do you understand your own personality: have you undertaken a personality profile test? Do the insights about your personality affect your career choice?
- What transferable skills do you have that might fit you for a different kind of career?
- How does your current work and life measure up to your inner values?
- What kind of roles and responsibilities do you prefer? Do you enjoy leading or following? Do you like to manage or be managed?
- What fears do you have that you need to overcome?
- What qualities do you have that you need to exploit or harness?

Your current job
- Do the features of your job fit with your personal style?
- How satisfied are you with your job – working hours, responsibility, location, patient contact, workload, income, challenge, opportunities for change or development, extent of socialising, your skills, on-call commitment, support from colleagues, variety?
- How satisfied are you with your career in general?
- What aspects of work do you value?
- Are there inner barriers that hinder your career advancement in your current job (e.g. self-doubt, low self-esteem)?
- Do you act the part in your post, even if you do not feel confident?
- Do you exceed your job description? You can impress others with your initiative and capability.
- Do you set yourself new targets within your job to keep your interest alive and provide new challenges?
- Do you nurture your relationships with other colleagues? You never know when you may need their support or help.

Looking outwards
- What opportunities are there in your current job for promotion or other roles or extending your skills?
- What opportunities might there be for developing new skills or enhancing current skills in your present job?
- What other jobs are on offer elsewhere for which you might apply?
- What other role(s) and responsibilities do you see yourself taking on?

continued opposite

- Have you got enough support from others at work?
- What qualities and skills do others perceive that you have?
- Is your potential recognised or realised in your current post?

Looking sideways
- How do your current workload and conditions impact on your family and other aspects of your non-working life?
- How satisfied are you with your lifestyle and the time spent outside work – sport, relaxation, hobbies, travel?
- How much quality time do you have for friends?
- What is the balance like between your current work and other aspects of your life?
- Do you have a mentor? A role model or influential colleague might well give your career a boost.

Summarise your results and form a conclusion.

Activity 7.2: Check your skills and strengths[1]

Tick the appropriate column in Table 7.1 to indicate whether you rate yourself as being competent in these areas at work; add any other items you think are important. Then tick the right-hand column to indicate which of the areas you have indicated *need attention*. Lastly, circle the areas that need attention that are a priority for you in your current post or are necessary to prepare for a career move. There may be other areas you want to add to the table as separate sections or as items within these 10 section headings.

Table 7.1: Self-assess your current skills – as a professional (and as an appraiser as relevant)[1]

	Competent	*Needs attention*
1 Personal effectiveness		
• decision making		
• negotiating		
• influencing		
• motivating others		
• winning commitment		
2 Personal management skills		
• time management		
• stress management		
• assertiveness		
• networking		
• delegation		
• presentation		
3 Clinical skills		
• basic as NHS professional		
• specialised for your job		
• new requirements (e.g. for new role or responsibilities)		
4 Practical skills		
• information technology		
• searching for evidence		
• health economics		
5 Being patient-centred		
• establishing relationships through sharing power, openness and honesty		
6 Organisational skills		
• clinical governance		
• patient involvement		
• public consultation		
• commissioning		
• health needs assessment		
• establishing new systems		
• implementing policies		
7 Social skills		
• influencing		
• communication		
• conflict management		
• leadership		
• change catalyst		
• relationship building		
• collaboration and co-operation		
• teamworking		
8 Special functions of your post		
• teaching		
• research		
• managerial		
• appraisal		

continued opposite

Table 7.1: *continued*

	Competent	Needs attention
9 Career attainment		
• qualifications		
• training		
• experience		
10 Social competence		
• empathy		
• understanding others		
• developing others		
• service orientation		
• working with and encouraging diversity		
• political awareness		

Activity 7.3: What changes do you want to make?

- To what extent are you content to remain in the same job or same practice or primary care organisation or other trust?
- To what extent will your current role satisfy you in one or three years' time?
- What is it that you most want to achieve? What are your career goals?
- Do your career goals conflict with other types of success or fulfilment that you are seeking in other areas of your life (for instance, financial goals, social goals, leisure goals, personal goals in relation to your family)?
- What resources do you have to help you achieve your career goals?
- Consider applying for promotion to show others that you are motivated to progress your career.

(i) Where do you want to be in ONE year's time? Write down your goals

Looking inwards

-

-

-

continued overleaf

Looking outwards

-

-

-

Looking sideways

-

-

-

Think widely: could you consider an academic career, research interest or audit, opportunities for teaching or mentoring, location, preferences or hobbies, alternative and parallel medical work, availability of cover by colleagues, supportive colleagues, sponsors and friends? Do you know of someone whose career you would like to emulate? If so, could you seek them out and ask them how they reached their post?

Build on your strengths and skills. Acquire new skills to develop your full potential. Taking on other roles and experience will add to your skills base. Skills developed outside work may be just as important as those developed as part of your job.

How will you know if you have been successful in achieving your goals?

(ii) Where do you want to be in THREE years' time? Write down your goals

Looking inwards

-

continued opposite

-

-

Looking outwards

-

-

-

Looking sideways

-

-

-

Activity 7.4: How are you going to get there?

Work out the series of steps you will need to take over the next 12 months to achieve your one-year goals; and longer-term action for your three-year goals. Think how to make things happen. To whom can you talk to get more information or advice? Who can you visit to see if their type of work appeals to you? Who can give you well-informed guidance or career counselling? How can you gain the preliminary achievements and experience that you need?

(i) Getting ready to make a change
What do you need to do first?
- Further reflection and review of how satisfied you are with your career, your job, your life in general – as in Stages 1 and 2 and 3

continued overleaf

- Discuss your satisfaction and options with others close to you – at home, your family and friends, work colleagues, trusted advisers and confidantes
- Find out more information and facts about other careers or new skills
- Ask someone for advice about opportunities in their field and what their jobs entail
- Seek careers guidance or career counselling from an impartial careers adviser
- Make a list of your options and reflect on their relative advantages

Are you ready to change?
- How positive are you about going ahead and making changes?
- Does what you are proposing fit with your ethics, values and boundaries?
- What is it that has limited you from making changes in the past? Have you overcome those constraints or barriers now?
- Are you clear about what interests and motivates you to work effectively?

So what will you do?

(ii) Make your plans happen with timetabled action
Think of:

- Setting goals
- What new insights, knowledge, skills and attitudes you need to develop
- Using your skills and experience
- Your timetable
- How you will proceed
- Support and resources you will need to make your plans come to fruition
- Overcoming limiting factors – what risks you need to manage
- Situations you may wish to influence – to prevent or provoke events or activities

So what will you do?

Activity 7.5: What will you do if you do not get the career development or progression that you want?

Write down your contingency plans. For instance:

- How could you change your current job so that you have more job satisfaction?
- Re-evaluate your options. What is your 'second choice' alternative career or new role?
- Re-assess your previous goals and objectives.
- What other skills might you develop within the NHS or in your leisure time?

continued opposite

- Could you get more balance into your life by building in more self-development time?
- Think if anyone else might help you through all your networks and contacts.
- Can you fit two different jobs into your life, working part time on each?
- Think again about what you really want out of life.
- Counter any self-defeating beliefs you possess.
- Institute better personal stress management.
- Build up your support – at work, with friends, with family and your partner at home.

Consider finding a mentor

A mentor might provide you with useful support in career planning and your career development. Or you might be a mentor for someone else and gain job satisfaction from that role.

A review of mentoring in relation to general medical practice described mentoring as 'a way of helping another understand more fully, and learn comprehensively from, their day to day experience'.[9] An enquiry into mentoring commissioned by the Department of Health defined mentoring as a 'process whereby an experienced, highly regarded, empathic person (the mentor), guides another individual (the mentee) in the development and re-examination of their own ideas, learning, and personal and professional development. The mentor, who often, but not necessarily works in the same organisation or field as the mentee, achieves this by listening and talking in confidence to the mentee.'[10]

In nursing and midwifery, the term 'mentor' can be used specifically to denote the role of the nurse, midwife or health visitor who facilitates learning and supervises and assesses students in the practice setting.[11]

Box 7.3:   Role of mentor from student nurse's perspective[12,13]

1 Supporter: give nurse advice, sort out problems or worries, be there as ally or friend
2 Guide and teacher: explain things, organise and arrange visits, be role model, feedback on performance to nurse
3 Supervisor: share problems, talk about mistakes and uncertainties, enable nurse to work out own solutions, allow gradual independence
4 Assessor: good understanding of assessment process and outcomes, implement assessment procedures

With increasing pressures on everyone's working day in the NHS it is vital to find new ways of coping and thriving at work. Mentoring supports professionals' growth in knowledge, skills, attributes and practice. Mentoring provides a confidential opportunity to share your feelings, express your views, test out ideas and raise questions. Having a mentor will allow you to take a step back and look at yourself, as a manager, as a leader, as a health professional or team player, and most importantly at you as a person.

Fostering a mentoring relationship develops, supports and equips staff with the skills they need to:

- support changes and improvements in patient care
- take advantage of wider care opportunities
- realise their potential.

References

1   Chambers R, Mohanna K and Field S (2000) *Opportunities and Options in Medical Careers.* Radcliffe Medical Press, Oxford.

2   Chambers R (1999) *Survival Skills for GPs.* Radcliffe Medical Press, Oxford.

3   Baldwin P (1999) *Cohort studies of Scottish medical school graduates.* In: First Oxford Conference on Medical Careers, Oxford University, Oxford.

4   Chambers R, Mohanna K and Chambers S (2003) *Survival Skills for Doctors and Their Families.* Radcliffe Medical Press, Oxford.

5   Department of Health (2003) *Job Evaluation Handbook.* Department of Health, London.

6   Department of Health (2003) *Agenda for Change. Proposed Agreement.* Department of Health, London.

7   Department of Health (2003) *NHS Knowledge and Skills Framework and Development Review Guidance. Version 6.* Department of Health, London.

8   Schein E (1996) *Career Anchors: discovering your real values.* Pfeiffer, Oxford.

9   Freeman R (1998) *Mentoring in General Practice.* Butterworth-Heinemann, Oxford.

10   Standing Committee on Postgraduate Medical and Dental Education (SCOPME) (1998) *Supporting Doctors and Dentists at Work. An Enquiry into Mentoring.* SCOPME, London.

11   English National Board for Nursing, Midwifery and Health Visiting and Department of Health (2001) *Preparation of Mentors and Teachers.* ENB, London.

12   Gray MA and Smith LN (2000) The qualities of an effective mentor from the student nurse's perspective: findings from a longitudinal qualitative study. *J Adv Nurs.* **32(6)**: 1542–9.

13   Gould D, Kelly D and Gouldstone L (2001) Preparing nurse managers to mentor students. *Nursing Standard.* **16(11)**: 39–42.

8

Evaluation and assessment of appraisal

Nationally there is as yet little guidance for organisations that wish to measure their performance or quality assure their appraisal system. You might find that some of the suggestions presented here are useful for you and your organisation and others seem impractical or less helpful in your circumstances. Feel free to adopt or adapt these ideas to suit you as you think how your appraisal programme – its content, delivery, processes and outcomes – can be evaluated. Consider whether the evaluation you choose will mirror the philosophy of the appraisal process.[1,2]

Evaluation is the act of examining and judging, concerning the worth, quantity, significance, quality, degree or condition of something. Evaluation may be approached from the perspectives of the individuals being appraised, the appraisers, programme or organisation. Reliability and validity are increased if several formats are used. Evaluation may include a combination of interview, participant observation and documentary analysis. Other methods of evaluation include completion of qualitative and quantitative marking schedules, peer review and observed practice.

Thinking about evaluation and assessment of the appraisal process

When you think about evaluating an appraisal programme, look at how well it achieves the aims set out for it. This is a step that requires careful consideration of what appraisal is for, from the perspectives of all key players. Evaluation is a systematic approach to the collection, analysis and interpretation of information about any aspect of conceptualisation, design, implementation and utility of appraisal programmes.

We may *assess* how individuals develop as a result of an appraisal and *assess* the appraisers to measure how well they have performed in their role. The *evaluation* measures how effective the appraisal process itself was in delivering any such development or change. Elements of both these aspects of assessment should be incorporated into an evaluation of an appraisal programme. In particular, the performance of appraisers may well be a key component in evaluating how well an appraisal programme trained those appraisers, for example. Ultimately, whether an individual member of staff's personal development is enhanced following an effective appraisal, with subsequent improvements in patient care, is a key factor to try to measure.

Having invested a lot of money into implementing appraisal in the NHS, the Department of Health may want to concentrate on the effectiveness of the completed appraisal programme, following all the changes required for the system to work. This is sometimes called a product or summative evaluation and is often carried out by independent observers. It is desirable to look at programme quality, usually during the earlier stages – sometimes called process or formative evaluation. This is often carried out by development personnel within an organisation, or even by key participants in the process, and includes feedback from those involved.

In this chapter we consider:

- evaluation from the perspective of those who are appraised
- evaluation from the appraiser's perspective
- evaluation from the trust, primary care organisation (PCO), Deanery or NHS perspective
- evaluation from the patient's perspective.

The evaluation cycle: outcomes of appraisal[3]

Evaluation is a vital component of the appraisal process. Like any monitoring process it is iterative. Without it we cannot improve and develop our systems or decide on the allocation of resources, and the professional development of personnel is more difficult. When we apply it to individual appraisal conversations, we often want to find out 'how the appraiser did'. When we apply it to programmes we often want to know 'Are we doing what we set out to do?' Because evaluation is cyclical, how it will be undertaken should be built in at the start of any new programme.

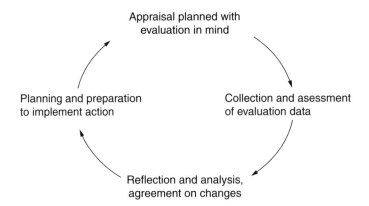

Figure 8.1:   The evaluation cycle.

Reflect for a moment on any aspect of your practice for which you have gathered evidence of your effectiveness. Consider the feedback you gather from participants, be they patients or others. At what stage are they asked for their comments? Does this give you time to respond to the issues they raise? Can their comments affect their experience or only that of those patients or others who follow? How often do you make changes in response to their comments? Do you get useful information back that helps you to make changes, either in the way you do things or in personal development? What sort of questions are you asking?

What about courses or educational programmes that you run? How do you know whether you are meeting your aims overall? What happens to those completing your courses. Are they performing better in the workplace? What could you do to increase the effectiveness of their learning experience?

Perhaps there are challenges and issues in society that the healthcare professions are not meeting. Could changes in our education and training programmes better fit up our trainees for the real world? How can we find that out?

For appraisal, the outcome we seek is increased effectiveness of healthcare professionals or others in the workforce, and ultimately improvements in patient care. Increasingly, as appraisal is implemented across the NHS workplace, we will need to seek evidence that it is robust, has been evaluated for performance and gives good value for money. In addition, with the link for doctors between appraisal and revalidation, the General Medical Council (GMC) and the public will seek reassurance that a quality-assured appraisal process has been evaluated for its ability to improve patient care. The model of evaluation as a cycle reminds us that the answers to questions we ask should inform developments that increase effectiveness. We need to seek information in a timely way so that improvements can be made as soon as appropriate. We need to critically analyse the information we get back to ensure that we respond to it in a direction that is likely to increase this effectiveness. Direct action needs to be taken before the cycle of appraisal is repeated.

Evaluation questions

So how do we know which aspects of appraisal are important to evaluate and what questions to ask? Kirkpatrick has described a hierarchy of evaluation, or four levels on which to focus questions.[4] These have recently been adapted for use in health education.[5] They can usefully be adapted for appraisal too. Table 8.1 considers the four levels that apply throughout the whole range of evaluative techniques and situations.

Table 8.1: Evaluating appraisal: the four levels[5]

Level	Evaluation of	Measure	Question
1	Reaction	Satisfaction or happiness	What is the participant's response to the appraisal programme?
2	Learning	Knowledge or skills acquired Modification of attitudes or perceptions	What did the participant learn?
3	Behaviour	Transfer of learning to workplace	Did the participant's learning affect his or her behaviour?
4	Results	Transfer or impact on society	Did changes in the participant's behaviour affect his or her organisation? Were any benefits or problems noted as a result of these changes?

These questions, at each level, can be asked of anyone involved in appraisal – those being appraised, appraisers or even patients – by changing the context or emphasis. Organisational outcomes are evaluated in just the same way.

Participant evaluation: appraiser and individuals who have been appraised

The commonest and quickest form of evaluation is to ask for feedback from those appraised or the appraiser. Many organisations have devised feedback forms that individuals complete after an appraisal conversation to comment on how useful they found the process. Feedback from appraisal evaluation forms such as this should help organisations to streamline their processes, monitor how individual appraisers are viewed by those they have appraised and make changes to ensure that the process is acceptable to participants.

Usual questions on such forms include: Did today meet your expectations? What aspects went well or did not go well? What helped this to happen or got in the way of a good appraisal for you? We can now see that these are Level 1 type of evaluative questions in the Kirkpatrick hierarchy.[4]

Sometimes the evaluation form will continue: what three things did you learn from your appraisal or what do you know now that you didn't know before? These are Level 2 type questions.

It is not common to be asked Levels 3 and 4 type questions, such as what things have you changed at work as a result of your appraisal, and what has been the impact of changes you have made? This is because these relate to delayed outcomes that cannot be evaluated on the day and will depend on effective completion of a well-planned and constructed personal development plan (PDP). Robust evaluation over time should aim to answer these higher-order outcomes.

What aspects might you ask an individual who has been appraised to evaluate?

Evaluative questions for those who are being appraised can be designed around the stages of the educational cycle of needs assessment → objectives setting → methods → assessment of outcomes, as described below.

Needs assessment

- Did your appraisal help you with relevant aspects of your practice?
- Were your needs met?
- What was the extent of needs that were not met?
- Were problems solved?
- What was the extent of problems still remaining?
- Were problems not tackled?

Objectives setting

- Was the objective of the appraisal made clear?
- What else did you need to know about?
- Was the organisational training or preparation for your appraisal appropriate?
- Was the organisational training or preparation for your appraisal helpful?

Methods
- Was the appraisal conversation well facilitated?
- Was the paperwork useful?
- Did you get the paperwork in time?

Outcomes
- Have you developed a meaningful PDP as a result of your appraisal session?
- Do you feel able to plan your personal development?

The opportunity to develop further following participant evaluation is sometimes limited by the quality or type of questions (or responses) focused on other issues – timetables, communications, sound, documentation, ambience and car parking. Sometimes the quality of the feedback reflects the level of insight those being appraised have into what a good appraisal experience would be like for them, the degree to which they are confident about making judgements about their appraiser, or some misunderstanding about the purpose of the evaluation questions and how it will affect them.

Leaving space for free text for comments can sometimes attract the best suggestions here. You will need to pose a question that is sufficiently inspiring to raise the level of the feedback. Consider using: *'What suggestions do you have to help appraisal really make an impact on patient care?'*

Remember that you do not have to evaluate everything! Sometimes you see evaluation forms that have attempted to evaluate every single aspect of appraisal using a very detailed questionnaire, several pages in length, with complex marking scales to be completed. This is rarely necessary. You want to find out about things you can change. After you have been using the same form for a while you should consider the type and amount of useful information you are getting and whether the questions need to be pruned or altered.

Characteristics of a good evaluation question for someone who has been appraised

These include being:

- appropriate: relevant to the point of appraisal
- intelligible: can be understood clearly
- unambiguous: means the same thing to all
- unbiased: does not trigger one response selectively
- simple: one idea only per question
- ethical
- pitched at higher levels on the Kirkpatrick hierarchy[2]
- valid: relates to what you think you are evaluating
- timely: asked at right time (e.g. not too soon if about application of learning or change).

Consider the evaluation form in Box 8.1 and to what extent it is a good example of a form that will produce meaningful information that can help development of appraisal for an organisation. (Actual evaluation forms are reproduced at the end of this chapter, which you may want to produce for use in your organisation.)

Box 8.1: Example of an evaluation form for an individual who is being appraised

Your thoughts and reflections on how your appraisal went will be valuable feedback for us as we develop the appraisal process.

Satisfaction
- Did your appraisal meet your expectations?
- What went well for you today?
- What could have gone better?

Knowledge and skills
- Did your appraiser help you effectively to consider your practice?
- What helped this to occur?
- What got in the way of this happening?

Transfer of skills
- What will you do differently in your everyday work or in preparing for appraisal next time?

Impact
- How will your professional development be affected by what you discussed in your appraisal?

The whole evaluation process should be valid, reliable, simple, practical and probably anonymous (you can offer anonymity to the person completing it or the person it is about – often the appraiser). Information about appraiser performance can be valuable if linked to a named appraiser, but individuals who have been appraised may be less frank in their feedback if they feel they will be identified.

Evaluations can be *quantitative* (numbers) or *qualitative* (descriptive) or both.[6,7] In a quantitative survey, you might be looking at:

- numbers of individuals who have been appraised who were satisfied with their appraiser
- numbers of completed appraisals per year
- reduction in patient complaints or resignations of healthcare professionals.

Or you could use qualitative techniques and seek to discover the subjective experience of those involved. Often these data will be gathered in free text form, maybe by interview with individuals, either on their own or in groups. Such data are extremely valuable, but the analytical techniques required to summarise them may be less familiar. A quantitative evaluation might focus on the numbers of completed PDPs – an easy statistic to gather – whereas a qualitative survey could ask individuals in what way their PDPs influenced their practice – information which is much less easy to gather and more complicated to summarise across a number of respondents. However, it may well be that the latter information is much more relevant to the purpose of appraisal.

Rating scales

These include Likert scales and semantic differential scales. The Likert scale is a popular scale used by sociologists and psychologists in research and can be applied in appraisal evaluation. It consists of an opinion statement followed by (usually) a five-point scale asking the respondent to indicate the extent to which they agree or disagree with that opinion statement. For example:

Please circle one of the numbers that best represents your view:

My appraiser really helped me to reflect on my practice   1   2   3   4   5

(1 = strongly disagree, through to 5 = strongly agree)

The semantic differential scale is somewhat different. Here a statement is given and the respondent is asked to rate it, usually on a seven-point scale with adjectives, such as *good–bad*, at either end of the scale. For example:

Please circle one of the numbers that best represents your view:

I felt that the amount of information from the PCO to help prepare for the appraisal was appropriate

1   2   3   4   5   6   7

(1 = bad, through to 7 = good)

Over a series of GP appraiser training workshops, participants were asked to identify useful markers for evaluating appraisal – these are given in Box 8.2.[8]

Box 8.2:   Ideas for evaluating appraisal from the perspective of those appraised

1   Straight after appraisal:

- The appraisal process: (i) how well organised all stages of appraisal process were, (ii) contentment with choice of appraiser, (iii) level of confidence in submitting information to primary care organisation, (iv) how clear the instructions were about the process, (v) how useful it was.
- Whether individual appraised perceived that there was time for reflection and planning in the appraisal session.
- Extent to which appraiser could answer questions about the appraisal process or the issues arising as part of the appraisal discussion.

continued overleaf

- Extent to which appraiser helped person appraised to: (i) reflect on practice, (ii) make plans, (iii) review career path, (iv) make changes, (v) resolve issues causing individual to be ineffective.
- Extent to which appraiser helped person to be: (i) comfortable with, (ii) trust – the appraisal process.

2 At six months/one year on:

- Extent to which action planned had been completed, and, if not, what had prevented it – in relation to learning, resources and practice.
- Comparisons of repeat learning or service needs assessment measures (e.g. 360° tool) show change (preferably improvement), how positive the individual felt in retrospect.
- Extent to which appraiser had helped individual they appraised to work more effectively: (i) as individual professional, (ii) as member of team.
- Whether GP appraised ultimately 'passed' revalidation without unexpected additional work.
- Number and type of complaints and comments from those appraised made to local professional committee or PCO or Deanery.
- Number of individuals appraised remaining in post anticipating appraisal process starting up, or after having an appraisal (i.e. were resignations triggered by fear of appraisal or other negative links to appraisal?).

Evaluation of personal development plans

In some ways the most tangible outcome of an individual's appraisal is the PDP, and this might also be the most relevant aspect to evaluate in terms of the quality of an appraisal conversation. To be truly effective, an evaluation tool needs to go beyond how many PDPs were completed to try and make a judgement about how appropriate the learning aims and methods were for a particular individual and whether any changes influenced patient care. Instructional aids for how to write or help facilitate the development of a PDP exist.[7,8] You can use these to build an evaluation tool for the effectiveness of that process. Consider the evaluation tool in Box 8.3, which is designed to be used after the appraisal has finished. Or see Appendix 3 for a brief checklist anyone can use to review the quality of a PDP. An organisation wishing to use this to evaluate this aspect of appraisal would additionally need to decide what 'score' would be acceptable, both for an individual appraised and across the organisation's appraisal programme.

Box 8.3:   Evaluation tool to measure the effectiveness of appraiser facilitation of a PDP[9]

There are four steps involved in the production of a PDP. The following questions help evaluate each stage:

Step One – Learning needs: *what does the individual most need to learn?*
Look for evidence that the appraiser carefully considered the information presented in the appraisal and helped to identify relevant learning needs in the light of this information.

continued opposite

Appraiser and individual being appraised agree that PDP objectives arise from the appraisal conversation	Yes/No
Some learning needs were present in a draft PDP	Yes/No
The learning needs will help with day-to-day work	Yes/No
The learning needs will help with self-esteem	Yes/No
The learning needs will help with career progression	Yes/No
Some learning needs address practice development issues	Yes/No
Some learning needs address patient/public needs or expectations	Yes/No
Some learning needs address local or national NHS priorities	Yes/No
Some learning needs will help this individual maintain fitness to practice	Yes/No
Other evidence (state):	

Step Two – Converting learning needs to objectives
The objectives should be SMART: **s**pecific, **m**easurable, **a**chieveable, **r**ealistic and **t**imed.

Step Three – Learning activities: *how will the individual best go about it?*
Look for evidence that the appraiser has considered what learning methods are most appropriate for this person and for these learning needs.

Information needs are addressed by reading and listening	Yes/No
Skills-based needs are addressed by observation and practice	Yes/No
Attitudinal development is addressed by discussing and analysing	Yes/No
The methods reflect previous learning methods chosen by this person	Yes/No
The methods fit with the resources of this person	Yes/No
The methods fit with the learning style of this person	Yes/No
These methods develop the person as a learner	Yes/No
The number and volume of learning activities is manageable	Yes/No

Step Four – Evidence of learning: *what will the individual put in the portfolio?*
Look for evidence that the appraiser has helped the person being appraised to identify appropriate examples of evidence that could demonstrate achievement for each set of learning needs and proposed methods.

The learner will keep a learning log	Yes/No
The learner will keep a reflective diary	Yes/No
Attendance certificates will show attendance at learning activities	Yes/No
Results of assessments after learning activities will be included	Yes/No
The individual appraised will self-evaluate change in performance after learning activities	Yes/No
The individual appraised will seek peer review evidence of change in performance	Yes/No
Learning will be shared with others in the workplace	Yes/No
A change in personal understanding will be documented	Yes/No
Audit will be carried out to document a change in practice	Yes/No

Group-based evaluation

In the NHS as a whole, many appraisers are new to the post and have limited experience. It is important that local appraiser groups are set up to support appraisers and share and develop best practice. A number of evaluation techniques work well in group settings and can enable the views of many to be shared. Round robins or snowball reviews are group-based evaluation methods that take participants through a number of formal steps during which their opinions and comments are elicited, shared, reviewed and compiled into a final list of strengths and weaknesses.[10] Either might work well in an appraiser workshop, where opinions are sought from all appraisers together about how the appraisal process was from their perspective – training and support aspects, for example.

Round robin evaluation

This is a method of eliciting, collating and rating every participant's most positive and negative comments about appraisal, as well as capturing their suggestions for improvement. The evaluation takes longer with more participants, although there is no theoretical maximum number who can take part. As an approximate guide, 30 people should take no more than 15 minutes to complete the evaluation, although they may need prompting to keep the pace up.

Ask each appraiser to write their most positive and most negative comments about the appraisals they have done at the top and halfway down one side of a filing card, respectively. If you have a very small number of participants, you might like to ask them to write their two most positive and negative comments to achieve a spread of concerns. On the reverse side of the card, ask for suggestions for improvement. Everyone should now pass their card to the person on their left, who should rate each comment on a scale of 1 to 5, 1 being 'strongly agree' and 5 being 'strongly disagree'. The cards should be passed on and rated in this way until each person receives his or her own card back.

The cards should then be collected, and the statements and their total and average scores collated into one document for feeding back to participants and contributors. The organisers of the appraisal system can also add a comment to the collated suggestions for improvement about which of these will be acted on and how.

The round robin method has the strength of allowing participants to express their own opinions, while determining how representative each individual's opinions are. The method has the possible weakness that it might not cover the evaluator's own particular concerns fully, but there is no reason why the evaluator should not join the circle and generate his or her own cards and statements.

Snowball review

To begin with, participating appraisers work alone, reflecting for a few minutes about their experiences of being an appraiser. In particular, each person should list what was especially good about it and what he or she would like to change about it. It is best if participants keep their lists to three good points and three suggestions for improvement. Participants should now form pairs and have open discussions to reach a composite list of good points and suggestions for improvement. At this stage, the list size could grow to four of each to accommodate divergent views. Neighbouring pairs should merge to form units of four and talk their way to a new composite list. Groups of four should now merge to form groups of eight to tackle the task of arriving at another list of composite views. Then one member from each eight should report their agreed conclusions to the whole group. Alternatively, you can collect one completed sheet from each group of eight and later collate the results and feed them back to those taking part.

The strength of the snowball method is that it involves all participants in contributing and discussing their views of appraisal. It also provides the opportunity for them to feed these back to those in the organisation who can influence how the system is run. Because it is a relatively time-consuming method however, the snowball review is best used for longer rather than shorter workshop sessions – perhaps an appraiser update training day. It can be used with groups of any size, but is particularly suitable as a way of ensuring the personal participation and contribution of all members of larger groups.

WWP: What Went Well, Why, Plan

This is another method that works well for appraiser workshops, to ensure full participation of all appraisers in the evaluation process. However, it can be applied to individuals who have been appraised working on their own or in pairs. Or one appraiser could appraise another and use the session for appraisal and mutual learning.

As a group-based evaluation method the participants reflect as a group, decide what went well, what went less well, decide why and then plan how things could be done better next time. It is particularly useful when group 'process' is being explored. If appraisers will be meeting over time to support each other, this is a good way to start. All appraisers, with or without a facilitator from the organisation, discuss what they thought went well. One of the group writes three headings across a flip chart:

What Went Well	Why	Plan

Members of the group list things they thought went well in column one. They then work out together why they thought each particular thing went well and list the reasons in column two. Then in the third column they write up a plan to follow next time they meet so they can build on what they have learnt. The next task is for the participants to decide together 'what went less well'.

The strengths of the WWP approach are that it is easy to do, requiring no special skills except the belief in the group's ability to work together. It is very enabling, making group members feel valued, in control and able to influence events. It also gives the group time for personal reflection about what they have gained individually from being an appraiser. It can indeed be used on an individual basis to evaluate appraisal, both for appraiser and those who have been appraised. The method has the possible weakness that a few strong members may influence the group, but good facilitation overcomes this. It does take some time, especially when the group is getting used to the method.

Ideas for evaluating the appraiser

Box 8.4 gives an overview of ideas gathered at a series of appraiser training workshops, describing useful markers for evaluating the appraiser.[8]

Box 8.4:   Ideas for evaluating the appraiser[8]

1   Self-assessment or self-report of appraisers in respect of:

- knowledge of resources available within PCO
- how appraisal went, how productive, how much covered, etc.
- contentment with timescale that appraisal portfolios sent in, prior to appraisal itself
- extent of information and balance of evidence of performance in others' appraisal portfolios
- extent of perceived support from PCO in arranging appraisals and feedback and other aspects of paperwork
- extent of perceived support from PCO in responding to practical/resource questions and issues arising from appraisals
- extent of perceived support from PCO in debriefing about pressures and strain on appraisers arising from appraisals
- extent of support for ongoing learning and development for appraisers from PCO
- satisfaction with PCO's establishment of underpinning/alternative referral processes for individuals with problems, in occupational health, assessment of performance, educational needs, career counselling
- extent to which appraiser felt sure of own role and boundaries.

2   Prediction of future performance of individuals appraised: (i) whether appraiser anticipated and discussed or (ii) recorded a problem that later arises.

3   Extent to which those appraised actively choose same appraiser next year, or actively refuse same appraiser next year, or frequency with which some appraisers are initially selected by individuals to be appraised.

4   Extent to which appraisers continue in their role in successive years.

5   Assessment of competence of appraiser: (i) peer review of appraisers' skills on ongoing basis (e.g. using video with informed permission, with third person observing with informed permission); (ii) self-assessed, e.g. against explicit competencies.

6   Ease of agreeing conclusion to appraisal in paperwork between appraisers/ individuals appraised (number that could not agree on final report).

7   Numbers of individuals appraised making appeals to PCO using official process or raising issues resolved at interim stage.

Peer review

Assessment of appraisers' performance by other appraisers could be an important future way to maintain quality in an appraisal system and may form an important part of an evaluation programme. Appraisers can be individually appraised to monitor quality. The challenge at the moment is that we do not have a readily available tool against which to measure performance. We do not know enough about what a good appraisal looks like.

There are processes in general practice training that look similar, which might be transferable and on which we can base an assessment tool for appraising the appraisers in future. Summative assessment of GP registrars and the membership of the Royal College of General Practitioners (MRCGP) examination have a consultation assessment by video element; and there is a tradition of video appraisal of GP trainers in action in a tutorial, for re-accreditation of training practices. In nurse training and education, there is a tradition of supervision and feedback that involves observation of actual practice, so the step to observation of appraisal for the training of appraisers might be a logical one.

Peer review of the teaching process itself, by having a colleague sit in and observe, is a well-established cornerstone of quality control in teaching institutions. As a method of personal and professional development for teachers it is a powerful tool and it can be a useful way to evaluate the effectiveness of a course. There are elements that can be borrowed from this experience to assess the competence of an appraiser.

Measuring what can be observed in the appraisal process and making judgements about efficacy are not easy tasks. You need to know what makes an appraisal effective (what criteria matter), how to discriminate between good and excellent practitioners (what standards to apply), and how to spot it happening (what tools are needed).

In the West Midlands Deanery, work is underway to develop and pilot a formative video assessment tool for appraisers (*see* Table 8.1). A video assessment tool allows observation of actual practice with the benefit of feedback that is directly informed by practice, rather than theory. It removes the observer from the intimacy of the appraisal conversation and keeps that conversation private at the time of the appraisal – with informed consent obtained from both parties, of course. Any such evaluation needs to stress that videoing is for training purposes, tapes will be securely stored, only be watched by those with an educational interest and will be destroyed after evaluation. If, at any time, the appraiser or the individual being appraised wants to stop the videoing, this should be respected.

Since any video assessment tool is in its infancy in deciding the important criteria, standards and tools required for observation and evaluation of an effective appraisal are best used as formative tools to aid appraiser development. Being subjective, it is unwise to consider their use as 'pass–fail' assessments of appraiser competence. The West Midlands tool comes complete with definitions of desirable skills but training and practice in their use will be needed before these can be reliably applied. At this stage detecting whether measures are present or absent is the extent of the judgement to be made.

A 'word picture' is given for each desirable skill, with examples that help both the appraiser in his or her preparation of a tape and the assessor in his or her assessment of the video tape.

A workbook with this information is given to the appraiser for completion and submission with his or her tape. The workbook would be used to highlight where each desirable skill has been demonstrated with formative advice. It remains confidential to the appraiser, although PCOs are aware that their appraisers have been through the process. This type of evaluation of appraisal might form part of the annual review, or appraisal, of appraisers.

Table 8.1: West Midlands video formative assessment tool for appraiser competence[11]

Listening: the appraiser demonstrates evidence of listening using such 'desirable skills' (DS) as

Present or absent

Active listening
Educational silence
Facilitating

Questioning: the appraiser demonstrates evidence of questioning to help the individual being appraised to become more focused and clear thinking using such DSs as:

Present or absent

Reflecting
Paired and open questions
Probing focused questions
Reflection space
Challenging (non-threatening)
Acknowledging success

Facilitating: the appraiser demonstrates evidence of facilitation to help the individual being appraised move forward using such DSs as:

Present or absent

Role modelling
Discussion of options
Sharing opportunities
Information giving
Negotiating skills
Direction
Knowledge of professional environment
Making judgements (non-judgementally)

Concluding: the appraiser demonstrates evidence of concluding the appraisal where the various strands of the discussion are brought together using such DSs as:

Present or absent

Feedback
Contracting
Housekeeping

Ambience: The appraiser demonstrates the active development of an ambience that facilitates the whole appraisal interview using such DSs as:

Present or absent

Non-judgemental
Supportive
Honest
Confidential
Encourages openness
Empathy
Talks as a colleague
Learner centred

Reproduced by kind permission of Dr Stephen Kelly, regional director of GP Education in the West Midlands.

Primary care organisation, or trust, or Deanery perspective

Others have warned that:

> In complex fields of practice there is a risk that [evaluation] highlights the readily measurable, over-emphasising detail, rather than promoting essential aspects of competence. In this way practice is trivialised through [evaluation] that fails to support competence development.[12]

Evaluation of appraisal is in danger of following the same route. It is challenging to consider what outcomes would reflect a 'good' appraisal process.

In the West Midlands Deanery, a model for the evaluation of appraisal is looking at appraiser training and its ability to prepare appraisers for the job. As such, it is a structure and process evaluation at lower levels on the Kirkpatrick hierarchy.[2] Outcome-based evaluations are harder to perform, and 'transfer' and 'impact' will be difficult to measure. The West Midlands evaluation project (*see* Table 8.2) does make a start and gathers much useful information that may influence future support and training provision.

Deaneries have been given the responsibility of assuring the quality of the NHS appraisal process. The questionnaire in Table 8.2 is designed to evaluate the experience of GP appraisers, their current training and their educational needs and development, in complete confidence.

Table 8.2: West Midlands Deanery appraisal evaluation tool[13]

Please complete or tick all appropriate box(es)

1	About you, the appraiser:		
1.1	Your gender	Male	☐
		Female	☐
1.2	Qualifying university/medical school	[..]	
1.3	Years in general practice (excluding time as GPR)	[..]	
1.4	Practice size (as number of partners)	[..]	
1.5	Are you a	GMS principal	☐
		PMS practitioner	☐
		Supplementary list GP	☐
1.6	Higher qualifications	MRCGP	☐
		MMEd Sci	☐
		DipMedEd	☐
		CertMedEd	☐
		Postgraduate Award	☐
		MRCP	☐
		FRCS	☐
		FRCGP	☐
		Other (please specify below)	
		[..]	

continued overleaf

Table 8.2: *continued*

1.7	Educational experience	Deanery GP tutor	☐
		PCT GP tutor	☐
		VTS course organiser	☐
		Undergraduate tutor	☐
		GP trainer	☐
		Other (please specify below)	☐
1.8	Do you work in a training practice?	Yes	☐
		No	☐
1.9	Have you had any prior experience of conducting appraisals?	Yes	☐
		No	☐
1.10	How many NHS GP appraisals have you conducted to date?	None yet	☐
		One	☐
		Two–four	☐
		Five–nine	☐
		Ten or more	☐
1.11	Please state your employing PCT as an appraiser	[..]	
2	About your selection and training:		
2.1	How were you selected?	Personal application (volunteer)	☐
		Approached directly by PCT	☐
		Applied for interview	☐
		Nomination [by whom ....]	☐
		Other (please specify)	
2.2	What initial training did you have?	Edgcumbe two-day	☐
		Edgcumbe one-day	☐
		RCGP two-day	☐
		RCGP one-day	☐
		Other (please specify) [............................]	☐
2.3	What further training sessions have you had?	None	☐
		PCT led by Deanery Appraisal Facilitator	☐
		Other (please specify)[............................]	☐

3   About your initial training

There is now a series of statements about GP appraisals and your training. Please circle the number which fits best with your personal experience about your training and appraisal abilities. These are all on a 1–6 scale.

1 means **strongly disagree**	2 means **disagree**	3 means slightly **disagree**
4 means **slightly agree**	5 means **agree**	6 means **strongly agree**

Please circle one number for each of these statements that best represents your personal view

continued opposite

Table 8.2: *continued*

		Disagree					Agree
3.1	After the initial training I understood the NHS GP appraisal process thoroughly	1	2	3	4	5	6
3.2	After the initial training I felt very confident to undertake my colleagues' appraisals	1	2	3	4	5	6
3.3	My training did not prepare me well to be an appraiser	1	2	3	4	5	6
3.4	After the initial training I knew what to do with all the forms	1	2	3	4	5	6
3.5	After training I felt less enthusiastic about being an appraiser	1	2	3	4	5	6
4	About your future training needs						
		Disagree					Agree
4.1	I need further help with learning how to handle unwilling and/or difficult individuals	1	2	3	4	5	6
4.2	I need further training in completing all the appraisal forms	1	2	3	4	5	6
4.3	I am prepared to sign off the appraisal personal development plan	1	2	3	4	5	6
4.4	I need more training to include educational theory before I could sign off PDPs	1	2	3	4	5	6
4.5	I need more information from the PCT to assist individuals accessing help and training	1	2	3	4	5	6
4.6	I would like to see a minimum list of evidence to be supplied by the individual being appraised	1	2	3	4	5	6
4.7	I feel fully prepared to undertake the appraisal of part-time and locum GPs	1	2	3	4	5	6
4.8	I would like more training about the particular problems of appraising supplementary list GPs	1	2	3	4	5	6
4.9	I think it is right that GP registrar appraisals should be conducted by other trained GPRs	1	2	3	4	5	6
5	Your views on appraisal so far						
		Disagree					Agree
5.1	The appraisal system in my PCT has has been very well organised	1	2	3	4	5	6
5.2	I have been impressed by my appraisal training	1	2	3	4	5	6

continued overleaf

Table 8.2:   *continued*

5.3	I think that PCTs are capable of running the appraisal process without any assistance from the Deanery	1	2	3	4	5	6
5.4	I think that the Deanery should be more involved in the co-ordination of the appraisal process	1	2	3	4	5	6
5.5	I think that appraisal should be kept as a developmental educational exercise	1	2	3	4	5	6
5.6	On the whole, those appraised have found their appraisals to be a worthwhile exercise	1	2	3	4	5	6
5.7	I am concerned that the revalidation appraisal link will demand a pass/fail result	1	2	3	4	5	6
5.8	If GPs had to 'pass' their appraisals I would resign as an appraiser	1	2	3	4	5	6

Other ideas for evaluating appraisal

At a series of appraiser training workshops, participants generated ideas as to how the NHS in general terms might evaluate appraisal (*see* Box 8.5).[8]

Box 8.5:   Ideas for evaluating appraisal from NHS perspective

- Number of appraisals undertaken as proportion of workforce working within PCO + numbers of appraisal forms returned (on time)
- Extent to which the PCO's learning agenda and business plans are informed by information derived from appraisals or individuals' PDPs.
- Extent to which quality specifications for competence of appraisers, the appraisal discussion, appraisal arrangements are fulfilled
- Records of changes arising from individual doctors' behaviour after appraisals or by completed PDPs enhancing the quality of individuals' practice or the quality of patient care in the wider NHS
- Extent of follow-up by appraisers of those being appraised in subsequent years
- Extent of initial and follow-up appraiser training and development available and taken up by established appraisers
- Extent to which training and support needs of appraisers in respect of appraisal are met by organisation
- Extent to which appraisals are assessed as being 'value for money' – indicators could be selected to reflect cost-effectiveness measures, e.g. changes in prescribing costs linked to appraisals
- Recruitment and retention in general in terms of numbers of health professionals and managers in PCO workforce – reflecting perception of appraisal and linked supportive culture of PCO
- Establishment of quality assurance framework for appraisal and systematic monitoring of framework and risks

---

An important component of an appraisal programme worth evaluating is the extent to which pooled and anonymised information is used to inform corporate planning or learning plans in a locality. Organisations vary greatly in the extent to which they have developed systems to enable this to happen effectively. At the very least the Department of Health expects that trusts and other PCOs will collate anonymous summaries of educational needs. Whether in a given area this then translates into educational provision is very patchy. The involvement of the views of healthcare practitioners in developing educational programmes would be a good-quality marker of the effectiveness of appraisal. Sophisticated organisations might have multi-disciplinary education teams that co-ordinate and organise learning opportunities for all groups of practitioners and managers, led by needs identified as recurrent themes in appraisals.

Patient perspective

From the perspective of the patient, an effective appraisal process is one that will ensure their safety, and will help keep healthcare practitioners and managers up to date and continuing to develop. Their views can be monitored as part of an evaluation that looks at numbers and nature of complaints from patients about health professionals and their performance, or by successive patient surveys.

There is currently increased interest in the self-regulatory activities of healthcare professions. Appraisal, as one component of a process that ensures practitioners are fit to practice, is coming under scrutiny and we need to ensure adherence to demonstrable quality indicators.

Conclusions

The General Medical Council states that it will not be appraisal per se but the robust, quality assurance processes within trusts and PCOs that will ensure the public continues to be served by a well-trained medical workforce. The test of that quality assurance will be in the outcomes of inspection and audit by the newly formed Healthcare Commission. The Health Professions Council and the Nursing and Midwifery Council have not made such a strong link between appraisal for their practitioners and regulatory accreditation, but all will be looking for a robust process that can deliver professional development.

We now need to be working on these quality assurance processes so that we know what we are evaluating appraisal against. Several questions still need addressing.

1   What are the competencies of an excellent appraiser?
2   Is it possible to measure the performance of an appraiser?
3   What does an excellent appraisal process look like within an organisation?
4   How can we evaluate appraisal? What are appropriate quality markers?
5   How can we be sure that appraisal will lead towards better patient care?[14]

We have started to address some of these questions here but some, especially the last one, are almost impossible to consider. The many ideas proposed for evaluation relate to the structure, process and outcomes of appraisal. Most need development to provide specific subjective and objective evidence; an evaluation framework might seek to triangulate evidence of effectiveness of different stages in the appraisal process from a variety of sources. Such measures of evaluation could be established once the PCO sets out its quality assurance framework for appraisal as part of its clinical governance system.

The Kirkpatrick's hierarchy would provide a good framework for NHS organisations to set out their approach to evaluation.[4] Evaluations uniformly set at Levels 1 and 2 would relate to the satisfaction of those involved with the process and knowledge and skills acquired, or the modification of their attitudes or perceptions. To make evaluation of appraisal as meaningful as possible, trusts, PCOs and/or Deaneries should aim at Levels 3 and 4 of Kirkpatrick's hierarchy focusing on behaviour and results, considering what things have changed as a result of appraisal, and the impact of the changes made. Nationally the relative contribution of trusts, PCOs and Deaneries in leading on and/or providing quality assurance for appraisal is not resolved. It is likely that responsibilities and roles will vary in different areas of the UK depending on local enthusiasm and capacity, unless there is strong national guidance soon.

Appraisal 'should be a vibrant, educational process'.[15] It should lead to focused professional development of healthcare practitioners and ultimately to improved outcomes for patients. Although the evidence is scarce, the one paper that looks closely at the link between patient care in a hospital setting and appraisal does show a positive link.[16] Outcomes are notoriously hard to link to inputs, however, and especially in healthcare there are a multitude of variables that might intervene between appraisal and healthcare improvement. It might be that at this stage the best we can develop are a series of process measurements. The NHS Clinical Governance Support Team and others involved in appraisal at a national level, feel that it is clinical governance that will drive improvements in patient care [17,18] and that we can rely on its implementation as a proxy marker of outcomes for patient care.

The sooner that the nature of the quality assurance framework is clarified, agreed and established on a national scale, the quicker we can develop a useful evaluation system for appraisal that is fit for purpose.

References

1 Rowntree D (1982) *Evaluation and Improvement*. PCP Educational Series, London.

2 Jayawickramarajah P (1992) How to evaluate educational programmes in the health professions. *Medical Teacher*. **14**: 159–65.

3 Wilkes M and Bligh J (1999) Evaluating educational interventions. *BMJ*. **318**: 1269–72.

4 Kirkpatrick D and Donald L (1994) *Evaluating Training Programs: the four levels*. Berrett-Koehler Publishers, San Francisco, CA.

5 Barr H, Freeth D and Hammick M (2000) *Evaluations of Interprofessional Education: a United Kingdom review of health and social care*. CAIPE/BERA, London.

6 Bowling A (1997) *Research Methods in Health. Investigating Health and Health Services*. Open University Press, Buckingham.

7 Bramley P (1996) *Evaluating Training*. Institute of Personnel and Development, London.

8 Chambers R, Tavabie A and See S (2003) Exploring ideas for the evaluation of the GP appraisal system. *Educ Prim Care*. **14(4)Supplement**: 579–83.

9 Hands S and Hughes M (2003) A tool to help GPs facilitate educational PDPs. *Educ Prim Care*. **14(4)Supplement**: 550–3.

10 Wakley G and Chambers R (2000) *Continuing Professional Development: making it happen.* Radcliffe Medical Press, Oxford.

11 James J, Mohanna K and Kelly S (2004) (personal communication). West Midlands Deanery Appraisal Support programme.

12 Grant J and Frances S (1999) *The Effectiveness of Continuing Professional Development.* Joint Centre for Education in Medicine, London.

13 Houghton G, Wall D and Kelly S (2004) (personal communication). West Midlands Deanery, Birmingham.

14 Mohanna K (ed.) (2003) Appraisal for GPs. *Educ Prim Care.* **14(4)Supplement**: 535–88.

15 Conlon M (2003) Appraisal: the catalyst of personal development. *BMJ.* **327**: 389–91.

16 West MA, Borrill C, Dawson J *et al.* (2002) The link between the management of employees and patient mortality in acute hospitals. *Int J Hum Res Manage.* **13**: 1299–310.

17 Scally G and Donaldson LJ (1998) Clinical governance and the drive for quality improvements in the new NHS in England. *BMJ.* **317**: 61–5.

18 Department of Health (2001) *Assuring the Quality of Medical Practice.* Department of Health, London.

9

Being an effective primary care organisation: using appraisal as a tool for continuing improvement

This chapter looks at what an effective organisation does in terms of structures, processes and outcomes to make the best use of appraisal as a team development tool. Trusts and other primary care organisations (PCOs) in the UK have a responsibility to make sure that the quality assurance processes behind appraisal are watertight. It is on these processes that the capacity of any appraisal system depends, to deliver an effective programme of continuing professional development (CPD) for all staff.

In some ways, the most important outcome for appraisal is the response of the organisation to the identification of unmet educational needs within its workforce. While it is clear that the responsibility to stay up to date and maintain fitness to practise remains an individual one, a healthy learning organisation will strive to provide a variety of learning opportunities, both in-house and by commissioning them from outside providers. These will be most effective if they are led by the needs identified through appraisal. Delivering a well-received, negotiated 'local learning plan' would be a good indicator of the effectiveness of the organisation.

The chapter is divided into three sections:

- resources necessary for effective appraisal
- systems and processes necessary within organisations for effective appraisal
- setting up a quality assurance framework for appraisal.

Resources necessary for effective appraisal

Resources necessary for effective appraisal processes include funding, available staff, staff development, educational expertise and provision of learning opportunities.[1]

Although being an appraiser builds on skills that many healthcare staff will already use in their day-to-day role, finding and training enough new appraisers has proved challenging in some areas. Training, updating and continuing development of appraisers will be important in maintaining a quality service. Ask the following questions in your organisation.

- What financial provision has been made for training appraisers and updating appraiser skills?
- Are commercial training bodies to be used or are there local providers of appraiser training?
- Are there local sources of expertise in training and development for ongoing appraiser support?

- Are appraiser support workshops funded and encouraged? If so, is there a designated lead?

To ensure the uninterrupted delivery of clinical care there will need to be arrangements to release those being appraised and appraisers for the dedicated time required for the appraisal. There should be information about back-fill arrangements or payments for sessional time or locums for both appraisers and those being appraised, or sessional appointments of appraisers and clinical staff to cover absent staff across the organisation. There should be provision to reconvene a further appraisal after postponing or halting an appraisal, e.g. if the person being appraised becomes distressed.

There should be occupational health support available for ill and distressed staff, those with alcohol or drug misuse problems and those whose physical or mental disabilities create functional problems. The appraisal process may well lead to increased identification of such problems. A responsible organisation will respond in a confidential, timely, appropriate and sensitive way once such needs have been highlighted. This may include individuals accessing existing support mechanisms, such as occupational health schemes in local hospitals, Relate or Alcoholics Anonymous, or may simply mean that all appraisers are trained to support and encourage others who are struggling to admit they need help and to contact their own GP.

Processes and resources are required for providing educational support for general or specific needs for appraisers and those they appraise. These should include a system for allocating or ring-fencing resources to address highlighted concerns relating to service development and delivery of care, to try and ensure the organisation is quick to respond with innovative educational events, for example. Such educational resources that already exist must be easily identifiable. You could survey all local providers of educational events, educational expertise or teaching and learning facilities to develop a database with contact details that appraisers can easily access when necessary. An organisation may well be able to commission and host good courses that already exist locally for its staff or, alternatively, devise educational events to meet staff needs. Gathering staff together with similar educational needs for local events will be more efficient than supporting individuals working and learning in isolation. Similarly, databases of books and learning resources such as simulators and on-line resources could usefully be catalogued and made accessible.

The nature and frequency of ongoing support for support and development of appraisers may include regular appraiser workshops to share best practice and discuss difficult appraisals, as well as peer review and appraisal of the appraisers themselves. Updating on changes in NHS policy, advanced skills training and refresher courses may also be needed. A local appraiser group may be convened with a chair or lead from within the group to organise such support and training.

Robust evaluation methods will have resource implications. Feedback should be gathered from the different perspectives described in Chapter 8 and fed into an evaluation system that can ensure best practice is applied. Personnel, time and money will be needed to do this well.

Systems and processes necessary within organisations for effective appraisal

Implementing an effective appraisal system across an organisation for the first time is a huge task. When the concept of clinical governance was introduced,[2] it was recognised that the learning culture within the NHS as a whole was fragile and needed nurturing.[3] The advice given then could equally well be adapted and applied to the aspects that need considering as we seek to achieve best practice with appraisal.

The following list should be a helpful start to organisations reviewing their appraisal processes.

1   Review the personal development needs of those managers and personnel charged with implementing appraisal. These might relate to:
   • management skills training to enable them to be effective
   • new knowledge and skills
   • their awareness of local and national policies
   • attitudes to various members of the multidisciplinary team.
2   Allocate lines of responsibility from leadership to delivery with clear expectations of what reports are required and when.
3   Assess support needs for all personnel and identify funding streams that will allow you to respond and provide resources to support appraisers and individuals who have been appraised.
4   Review and realign priorities in allocating resources so that your organisation can respond to educational needs of the workforce, identified through appraisal.
5   Identify and develop links with all key local figures in the provision of educational activities.
6   Continue to clarify and promote the organisation's strategies so that staff learning plans can be aligned with local priorities.
7   Devise ways to inform healthcare practitioners about local indicators of health, such as:
   • making anonymised morbidity and mortality data and practice-specific indicators of performance widely available, to underpin the appraisal process
   • enhancing IT infrastructure and support to achieve reliable and accurate data
   • disseminating regional and national directives to inform practitioners' work.
8   Consider how you might marry the education and training resources and activities in your organisation with the needs of staff and the health needs of the local population. You might:
   • undertake a locality health needs assessment seeking the advice of those in public health, local government and the public
   • map out the numbers and balance of the workforce
   • identify a central figure to collate recurrent themes from anonymised learning plans across the organisation.

At a series of appraiser training workshops, appraisers were asked to identify what aspects of management support for appraisal they felt were important.[1] Some of these suggestions fit well with a checklist style quality assurance approach, and are listed in Box 9.1.

Box 9.1:   Checklist for an effective appraisal process

An organisation will:

1   have a standard contract for all appraisers
2   have a fair method of allocation of appraisers to individuals to be appraised
3   have a universal agreement about the confidential status of information obtained from appraisals
4   provide guidance as to the balance between maintaining confidentiality and seeking the advice of others about the contents of the appraisal discussion (such as when risk to patient safety is suspected)
5   have explicit protocols for involving others when an appraiser has evidence that patient safety is at risk informed by whether the individual being appraised shows insight or not
6   develop transparent and locally known parallel processes for poor or under-performance of healthcare professionals in cases where appraisal needs to be terminated
7   have a clear and accessible complaints system for those being appraised with a named person responsible for managing such complaints and a protocol for acting on complaints received
8   make a guarantee of indemnity for appraisers where the person having been appraised makes an official complaint. Include information about the explicit limits of that indemnity
9   outline the expected action if an appraiser is found to be incompetent following a complaint from someone who has been appraised, or other form of notification
10   develop guidance on standard setting in relation to expectations of depth and scope of appraisal portfolios and the contribution of an individual member of staff to the local health economy and the wider NHS
11   evaluate the performance and practice of appraisers
12   define the extent of flexibility permitted in arranging appraisal discussions, e.g. setting for appraisal discussion in health, educational or leisure venues; time period for completing associated paperwork, etc.
13   decide on and standardise the amount and type of centrally available performance data that will be forwarded to those being appraised to help them to reflect on their performance
14   have a clear strategy for pooling anonymised information from appraisals to influence policy/development and for resources allocation
15   develop a 'trouble-shooting guide' with lists of people or other sources of help to consult if there are problems relating to any of the above.

Setting up a quality assurance framework for appraisal

One way to quality assure appraisal is to have 'second-tier' or third-party educational or managerial supervision that can oversee or advise on the process. For example, for doctors and dentists, Deaneries could:

- assume a role in developing an overarching policy on the standards required of educational providers, and a process of review and evaluation of all such provision
- provide or administer a quality assurance framework for all appraisal process within PCOs, maintaining uniformity across all PCOs in region, and liaise with other Deaneries across the UK
- ensure that overlap of all accrediting/appraising processes of GPs and dentists, trainers, course organisers, etc., is synchronised with appraisal/revalidation systems and structures
- provide a resource bank to help those with educational and skill needs identified by appraisal
- lead on the provision of ongoing training and development support for GP and dentist appraisers, e.g. setting the curriculum and quality standards.

In the West Midlands region, work is ongoing to develop a self-assessment quality assurance framework in the form of a 'toolkit' that will be available to all PCOs to help them look at how they are performing on appraisal. It includes suggestions and examples of good practice gathered from around the region and nationally, checklists to evaluate the effectiveness of different aspects of structure and process, examples of evaluation tools and appraiser development tools. It is intended to be used alongside the evaluation tools described in Chapter 8. The actual toolkit takes the form of a lever-arch file with examples and suggestions of the type of forms and systems that might be used, under each heading (*see* Box 9.2). For other organisations considering developing such a toolkit there are likely to be local tools that could be collated under these same chapter headings.

Box 9.2: Quality assurance toolkit for a PCO's self-assessment of the appraisal process

This toolkit is designed to look at management structures and processes. It includes forms, ideas and suggestions that you may want to use to look closely at how well appraisal is managed in your organisation. An effective organisation will have locally relevant evidence in each section. It is not a compulsory exercise, and the criteria in each 'chapter' are suggestions or recommendations only, but as you work towards completing each chapter you will find ideas that will help you to evaluate what you are doing and enable you to compare your performance with suggestions from other organisations.

Section 1: Training, information and communication
1   There will be a clear statement of the role and philosophy of appraisal as a developmental process and its place within the organisation

continued overleaf

---

2 An effective educational programme should be developed for communicating to all staff the aims and objectives of appraisal as a formative, developmental process
3 There should be an overall statement of who should participate in appraisal training: e.g. GP principals and non-principals, practice managers. All PCO managers involved in the process of appraisal should have this training
4 Ensure you have a well-functioning information system in place. The PCO should aspire to be in email contact with all practices and all appraisers
5 Develop a policy describing how ongoing appraiser training needs will be met, with a named person responsible for training and development and identification of adequate resources
6 Develop a policy describing how ongoing information needs of those appraised will be met, with a named person responsible for training and development and identification of adequate resources
7 Devise, and disseminate to all participants, a flow chart documenting practical aspects of appraisal information sharing, such as a clear statement about the use of electronic or paper appraisal forms, who is to fill them out and at which stage, for what purposes they will be used, where they will be sent and how confidentiality will be maintained
8 An appraisal workshop should be set up, and adequately resourced, for support and development of appraisers, with a lead identified from within that group

Section 2: Management and administration
1 There should be a corporate understanding that appraisal must be adequately resourced with structures in place to describe the funding arrangements and ensure they persist
2 There should be a named educational lead for appraisal, with responsibility at strategic level, who sits on the professional executive committee, or equivalent in PCOs
3 There should be a trained administrator with overall responsibility for all practical aspects of implementing appraisal
4 There should be a clear statement about how appraisers and those to be appraised will be matched, how much choice is allowed, whose responsibility it is to set up appraisal meetings and who will collate the paperwork
5 It should be decided whether and how centrally available pre-appraisal data will be supplied to individuals awaiting appraisal, e.g. prescribing or immunisation data and the status of this information, i.e. if it is formative to aid personal reflection
6 A policy on action to be taken in the event of the individual being appraised or the appraiser not complying with this process should be decided and disseminated, e.g. who should chase up those booked for appraisal who fail to submit the completed forms on time
7 The process of activating payments for sessional time to the appraiser and individuals appraised following the appraisal meeting must be clear (if appropriate)
8 A feedback form to gather the views of those appraised should be available after each appraisal with clear instructions on when and how this is to be completed and returned

continued opposite

Section 3: Appraiser quality

1 There will be an appropriate, locally negotiated job description for appraisal appointments
2 There will be a person specification for appraiser appointments specifying required and desirable characteristics
3 Appraisers will be appointed on the basis of the application form and interview, assessing their suitability against the pre-defined person specification
4 All appraisers will sign a contract specifying their roles, responsibilities, terms and conditions of the post
5 All appraisers will undergo sufficient, appropriate training before starting to appraise, and updating thereafter to enable them to perform well
6 Educational appraisal of the appraisers will be carried out by peer review in a mutually supportive appraisal workshop
7 Educational evaluation of the appraisal process itself will be carried out and used to inform the future development of appraisers
8 Continuing professional development of appraisers will be addressed under the guidance of the PCO education lead or local education experts as agreed, and this will be built into the PDPs of all appraisers
9 Criteria by which underperformance of appraisers will be assessed will be locally agreed and there will be a transparent de-selection process

Section 4: Ensuring the educational quality of appraisal

1 Appraisers will be trained in the art of creating educational objectives from identified needs and facilitating an educational PDP
2 PDPs will be developed according to sound educational principles and training, and updating in those principles for appraisers will be given where appropriate
3 There will be an evaluation tool for reviewing the effectiveness of PDPs
4 There will be a safe and effective system for gathering and confidentially storing the outcomes of appraisal, e.g. 'Form 4' for doctors
5 A named person, probably a clinician, will be responsible for collating, anonymising and summarising the educational needs identified in these outcome data. Recurrent themes arising in appraisals throughout the PCO will be used annually to inform the educational strategy for the organisation
6 Consideration will be given to how educational provision will be provided and resourced, e.g. protected learning time initiatives, PCO training and development or commissioning of courses, staff education and development budgets
7 So far as it is possible and robust systems exist to do so, there will be an annual evaluation of the appraisal process as it affects all participants, including satisfaction, acquisition of knowledge and skills, transfer of learning into the workplace and assessments of the impact of educational development. Information from this evaluation will in turn feed into the education strategy for subsequent years

Reproduced with permission of the West Midlands Regional Director of GP Education[4]

Summary

Only three aspects are essential to ensure an effective appraisal system in any organisation. If you can answer 'yes' to the following three questions, the chances are that you have an effective appraisal process.

1 Is there a named person with overall responsibility, enthusiasm and dedicated funding to ensure that appraisal happens?
2 Is someone responsible for collating all recurrent themes in the educational needs that are identified in the appraisals across the workforce and making a plan to meet them?
3 Is there a workshop for support and development of appraisers?

Much of the advice and many of the suggestions in this chapter are subsets of these three questions. They flow from them and will themselves be triggered if these three aspects are attended to. However, like any other new process, appraisal for those in the NHS is taking time to 'bed in'. Until we achieve a level of confidence and competence in implementing appraisal, these checklists will help organisations make it as effective as possible.

References

1 Chambers R, Tavabie A and See S (2003) Processes and systems that GP appraisers expect primary care organisations and deaneries to set up in relation to appraisal. *Educ Prim Care.* **14(4) Supplement**: 584–6.
2 Department of Health (1997) *The New NHS: modern, dependable.* The Stationery Office, London.
3 Wakley G, Chambers R and Field S (2000) *Continuing Professional Development in Primary Care: making it happen.* Radcliffe Medical Press, Oxford.
4 Dhaliwal J, Mohanna K and Kelly S (2004) (personal communication). West Midlands Deanery Appraisal Support programme.

APPENDIX 1

Template for a job description and person specification of an appraiser, based on the NHS Knowledge and Skills Framework[1]

1 General details
Job title: Appraiser
Location: Base: PCO
Time commitment: A minimum of X appraisals within 12-month period
Salary: Agreed PCO pay scale (if independent contractor) or within main job role
Additional allowances: Travel, training, etc.
Tenure: Fixed term (e.g. 2 years)

2 Relationships
Responsible to: Clinical governance lead in the PCO

3 Main purpose
To undertake appraisals of XX staff in accordance with guidance from the Department of Health and professional registration bodies.

4 Declaration
The appraiser must make a declaration at appointment (and if a pertinent situation occurs while in post) that he or she is not currently under investigation for any criminal offence or local complaints or disciplinary procedure, which might bring the appraisal process into disrepute.

5 Core competencies
Communication skills: consistently practise good communication skills.
Personal and people development: develop own and others' knowledge and practice across professional and organisational boundaries in relation to appraisal.
Health and safety and security: promote others' health, safety and security in relation to appraisal.
Service development: develop and improve NHS services through appraisal process.
Quality improvement: demonstrate personal commitment to quality improvement, offering others advice and support as an integral part of the appraisal process.
Equality, diversity and rights: enable others to exercise their rights and promote equal opportunities and diversity, through appraisal.
Promotion of self-care and peer support: encourage others to promote their own current and future health and wellbeing, through appraisal.

Ability to manage the appraisal process: process and manage data and information and maintain confidentiality.

Ability to carry out needs assessment: interpret, appraise and synthesise data and information appropriately, within the appraisal process.

Ability to contribute to and/or co-ordinate the support system for appraisal process: develop and sustain partnership working with those appraised, practice, PCO and Deanery (as relevant).

Leadership skills: lead others in the development of knowledge, ideas and work practice as integral part of appraisal process.

Protected time: identify and negotiate protected time to devote to appraisal process, follow-up action plans and take active part in local learning sets for peer appraisal and support.

6 Person sought

As an appraiser your prime focus should be to deliver better healthcare for patients by assisting your colleagues in their personal development. You will need to develop the trust and respect of those you appraise in order to facilitate their openness and honesty in discussing with you their successes and difficulties. You will need to recognise and challenge your own values and prejudices and bring an open mind to each appraisal. You will need to listen, be able to sincerely congratulate, and also challenge and explore difficult and sensitive issues. You will then need to be able to negotiate a mutually acceptable, realistic action plan which will provide those you appraise with a 'road map' to their professional future. You will need to do all of this honestly and in good faith so as to be able to sincerely sign that the resulting paperwork and outcomes are robust enough to contribute to the quality assurance process of your organisation or a professional body. All this will give you considerable professional satisfaction.

Date job description revised 18-7-04

Variation to job description
The XX PCO reserves the right to vary the duties and responsibilities of its employees within the general conditions of the scheme of pay and conditions and employment-related matters. Thus it must be appreciated that the duties and responsibilities outlined above may be altered as the changing needs of the service may require.

Employment specification/Interviewee assessment form
PCT: Post title: Appraiser (e.g. GP appraiser)   Date:

Essential (E) /Desirable (D) factors for post Please tick as appropriate			*Assessment/notes*
A Education:	E	D	
Medical degree	✔		
Qualified as GP (accredited as GP by JCPTGP)	✔		
MRCGP		✔	
Satisfactory completion of GP appraiser training	✔		
B Experience:			
Worked as a GP for minimum of three years	✔		
Works as GP currently or within previous two years	✔		
Background in training and development		✔	
C Specific skills, aptitudes and knowledge:	E	D	
Local knowledge of the area		✔	
Communication skills	✔		
Development of personal/people development	✔		
Health and safety and security	✔		
Service development: patients, appraisal process	✔		
Quality improvement	✔		
Equality, diversity and rights	✔		
Promotion of self-care and peer support	✔		
Data processing and management of appraisal process	✔		
Carrying out of needs assessment	✔		
Coordination of support system for appraisal process	✔		
Leadership skills	✔		
D Personal qualities:			
Credible with other GPs	✔		
E Can create protected time for appraisal	✔		
F Health/physical abilities:	E	D	
Physically and psychologically capable of undertaking the work of GP appraiser	✔		

Overall assessment/general comment
Completed by:

Reference

1   Chambers R, See S, Tavabie A and Hughes S (2004) Composing a competency based job description for general practice appraisers using the NHS Knowledge and Skills Framework. *Educ Prim Care*. **15**: 15–29.

APPENDIX 2

Example of a template for your personal professional development plan – start with one main topic and build others on as you justify needing to learn more about them

(Reproduced with permission from Wakley G and Chambers R (2000) *Continuing Professional Development: making it happen.* Radcliffe Medical Press, Oxford)

- What topic?

- Justify why topic is a priority:

  A personal and professional priority.

  A practice or workplace priority.

  A district priority.

  A national priority.

- Who will be included in your personal plan? (Anyone other than you – doctors, members of your team, patients?)

- What baseline information will you collect and how?

- How will you identify your learning needs? How will you obtain this and who will do it: self-completion checklists, discussion, appraisal, audit, patient feedback?

- What are the learning needs for your department or practice and how do they match your needs?

- Any patient or public input to your personal development plan?

- Map your learning needs against the 22 core and specific dimensions of the KSF:

  Communication

  Personal and people development

  Health, safety and security

  Service development

  Quality

  Equality, diversity and rights

  Assessment of health and wellbeing needs

  Addressing individuals' health and wellbeing needs

  Improvement of health and wellbeing

  Protection of health and wellbeing

  Logistics

Data processing and management

Production and communication of information and knowledge

Facilities maintenance and management

Design and production of equipment, devices and visual records

Biomedical investigation and reporting

Measuring, monitoring and treating physiological conditions through the application of specific technologies

Partnership

Leadership

Management of people

Management of physical and/or financial resources

Research and development

- Objectives of your personal development plan arising from the preliminary data-gathering exercise

- Action plan (include timetabled action, expected outcomes)

- How does your personal development plan tie in with your other strategic plans?

- What additional resources will you require to execute your plan and from where do you hope to obtain them? (Will you have to pay any course fees? Will you be able to organise any protected time for learning in working hours?)

- How will you evaluate your personal development plan?

- How will you know when you have achieved your objectives? (How will you measure success?)

- How will you disseminate the learning from your plan to the rest of your team and patients? How will you sustain your new-found knowledge or skills?

- How will you handle new learning requirements as they crop up?

Record of your learning: write in topic, date, time spent, type of learning

	Activity 1	Activity 2	Activity 3
In-house formal learning			
External courses			
Informal and personal			
Qualifications and/or experience gained?			

APPENDIX 3

Structured review of the quality of the personal development plan*

* This PDP review tool has been developed from various initiatives including the PDP assessment tool of the Eastern Deanery and the APD assessment tool of the Royal College of General Practitioners.

Criteria	Level C	Level B	Level A
Step 1 Assessed and prioritised learning needs	Some attempt to identify and/or prioritise personal learning needs, but subjective rather than objective approach	Good attempt to identify and prioritise personal learning needs, by range of subjective and objective methods	Systematic approach to identifying and prioritising personal learning needs, by wide range of subjective and objective methods
Step 2 Defined learning objectives	Objectives for learning plan loosely related to learning needs	Objectives for learning plan are specific and relevant to learning needs	Objectives for learning plan are specific and justified by learning needs; they show insight into potential improvement in performance
Step 3 Undertake learning plan	Learning plan is simple outline, loosely related to prioritised learning needs *and* type of learning methods may not be appropriate for learning needs	Timed learning plan is relevant to prioritised learning needs *and* type of learning methods are practicable and appropriate for learning needs	Timed learning plan is detailed and relevant to prioritised learning needs *and* type of learning methods are appropriate for learning needs and maximising learning opportunities
Step 4 Evidence of learning planned at last review and relevant change in performance	Little evidence of reflection on, or evaluation of, *overall* learning and achievements Limited attempt to assess performance in a few areas, with limited evidence of improvement(s) in performance	Some evaluation of learning and achievements by method that is appropriate for purpose Some reflection on extent to which learning needs have been met and what is yet to be learned Reasonable review of performance with some evidence of improvement(s) in performance	Robust evaluation of learning and achievements by at least one objective method that is appropriate for purpose Detailed reflections on extent to which learning needs have been met and what is yet to be learned Systematic review of performance with evidence of significant improvement(s) in performance

You might decide on a **scoring policy**. For instance, you might award a total of 12 points for an excellent PDP which merits full marks by earning a Level A score for each of the four steps. If the review of the PDP for a particular step:

- does not reach Level C, the score for that step would be 0
- is Level C, the score for that step would be 1
- is Level B, the score for that step would be 2
- is Level A, the score for that step would be 3.

APPENDIX 4

Example of an honorary contract for independent contractor (e.g. GP, dentist, pharmacist, optometrist) acting as appraiser for a primary care organisation: statement of terms and conditions

(Adapted from Wolverhampton City Primary Care Trust (2002) *GP Appraisal Toolkit*)

(*Insert name of locality*) aims to provide high-quality services to people who need treatment, care or advice. It aims for its services to be effective, responsive and friendly. The primary care organisation (PCO) expects all its employees to support and enhance its care and overall quality of service. It also expects each of its staff to act in a way to justify public confidence and enhance the good reputation of (*insert name of locality*).

Personal

Name:
Address:
Appointment: Appraiser
Service or area: Clinical governance
Date of appointment: (insert start date)
Review date: (insert review date)
Remuneration: (insert terms)

Services to be provided by the appraiser

So long as s/he shall continue to service (*insert name of locality*) under the terms of this agreement the appraiser will undertake the appraisal programme outlined below.

- Prepare for appraisal and agree the agenda with each individual to be appraised.
- Ensure that each appraisal is conducted in line with the PCO/DoH guidance.
- Support each person appraised in considering their practice over the last year.
- Agree objectives and the key elements of a personal development plan (PDP) with each individual appraised, except in circumstances where the person disagrees with the appraisal and an appeal is being raised.

- Agree actions with the PCO required to support the individual to meet their objectives and fulfil their PDP.
- (If GP appraisal) Discuss progress made by each GP appraised towards revalidation (and assist with any overview required after five years for the GMC revalidation folder).
- Record appraisal outcomes and convey them to the clinical governance lead.
- Maintain confidentiality over the detail of appraisal discussions.
- Attempt to build positive working relationships with the individual appraised and follow up appraisal discussions to review progress at least once during the following year as appropriate.
- Identify, where possible, any early warning signs that an individual may be in difficulties and agree with the individual how this can be dealt with.
- In exceptional circumstances, if seriously deficient or dangerous practice is encountered, refer in line with local procedures (remaining mindful of overriding individual professional duties in relation to the performance of colleagues).

To be provided by the PCO

- Contact details will be provided by the clinical governance team in order for the appraiser and those being appraised to liaise and agree appraisal dates.
- Paperwork will be sent to those being appraised at least two months prior to the appraisal.
- The appraisal venue will be agreed between appraiser and those being appraised.
- Dates for reviews will be arranged between appraiser and individuals being appraised.
- Training for appraisers will be arranged by the PCO and associated expenses incurred by appraisers reimbursed.
- Consideration will be given to supporting reasonable actions required by those being appraised to meet their objectives and fulfil personal development.

Notice period

Either side should give three months' notice of their intention to terminate this arrangement.

Health and safety

The PCO has an obligation under the Health and Safety at Work Act 1974 to provide safe and healthy working conditions. You are required to co-operate with management in discharging its responsibilities under the Act and to take reasonable care for the health and safety of yourself and others.

Personal property

The PCO advises its staff that responsibility is not accepted for articles lost or damaged on the PCO's premises, whether by fire, theft or otherwise, with the exception of money or valuables that have been handed to the PCO for safe custody and for which a receipt has been given.

Confidentiality

Information concerning patients and staff is confidential and must not be disclosed to any unauthorised persons. In instances where it is found that a member of staff has disclosed any such information this could result in disciplinary action being taken against them. The Data Protection Act 1984 also renders an individual liable for prosecution in the event of unauthorised disclosure of electronically stored information. A breach of confidence could also result in civil action for damages.

Equal opportunities

You are advised at all times to carry out your responsibilities with due regard to the PCO's Equal Opportunities Policy.

Conflict of interest

In accordance with the Codes of Conduct and Accountability you must declare to the PCO any financial interest or relation you may have which may affect the PCO's policy or decisions.

Indemnity

(*Name of locality*) will take responsibility for all your actions in the course of the appraiser's duties under or in connection with this agreement, other than those involving bad faith, wilful default or gross negligence.

Signed ....
(*for the locality*)

Date ....

Acceptance

I accept the terms and conditions as set out in this letter of appointment

Signed ....

Date ....

APPENDIX 5

Sources of help in relation to appraisal

Websites

- American College of Physicians and American Society of Internal Medicine (includes diagnosis aids)
  www.acponline.org/public/bedside/?idx
- British Association of Medical Managers
  www.bamm.co.uk
- British Medical Association (BMA)
  www.bma.org.uk/ap.nsf/Content/_Home_Public
- Clinical Governance Support Team
  www.cgsupport.nhs.uk
  www.gpappraisal.nhs.uk
- Edgecumbe Consulting Group Ltd
  www.edgecumbe.com
- General Medical Council (GMC)
  www.gmc-uk.org/revalidation/index.htm
- Health Matters Online
  http://health.mattersonline.net
- National electronic Library of Health
  www.nelh.nhs.uk
- NHS appraisals toolkit (Sowerby Centre for Health Informatics at Newcastle [SCHIN])
  www.appraisals.nhs.uk
- Royal College of General Practitioners (RCGP)
  www.rcgp.org.uk
- School of Health and Related Research (ScHARR)
  www.shef.ac.uk/~scharr
- TRIP database
  www.tripdatabase.com

- Educational Appraisal Skills – an interactive programme for trainees and trainers www.appraisal-skills.nhs.uk
  This is an online educational package that has been developed to provide medical trainers and trainees in hospital medicine and in general practice with the opportunity to use Web-based technology to help develop their skills in appraisal.
- Performance Appraisal Services www.performanceappraisal.co.uk
  The site of a UK company that provides performance appraisal services. The site gives a selection of performance appraisal articles covering a wide range of issues, such as aims, purpose of developmental performance appraisal, and what if it did not exist.
- Appraisal and Revalidation www.appraisaluk.info, www.revalidationuk.info

This site is a joint initiative of the General Medical Council and the Department of Health. It has a number of articles written by doctors on the appraisal process, such as 'Ten ways to get the most out of your appraisal'.

* Department of Health www.dh.gov.uk/PolicyAndGuidance/HumanResourcesAnd Training/LearningAndPersonalDevelopment/Appraisals/fs/en
  This site gives access to all relevant guidance and appraisal forms for consultants, GPs, non-career-grade doctors, etc.
* Electronic Journal of Sociology www.sociology.org/content/vol005.001/coates.html
  Article using a case study to discuss the experience in a trust hospital.
* Health Matters Online http://health.mattersonline.net
  A resource for health professionals to find ways to show that they are competent in their clinical work.
* Royal College of Obstetricians and Gynaecologists www.rcog.org.uk
* Cyber Medical College www.cybermedicalcollege.com/CPDPortfolio/AppraisalToolkit
  This is a website offering free online healthcare education and training.
* General Medical Council www.gmc-uk.org
  Information on revalidation and appraisal.

Index

Page numbers in *italics* refer to tables or illustrations

accreditation, using university frameworks
    for documenting prior learning
    120–1
Accredited for Prior Experiential Learning
    (APEL) 121
administration of appraisal schemes *172*
Agenda for Change initiative 57–9, *58*,
    133–4
    see also Knowledge and Skills Framework
aims of appraisal schemes 3–4, 164
    see also organisational (PCO) objectives
analysis and framework tools for PDP
    79–83, 178–81
    and evaluation checklists *152–3*
    use of degree/postgraduate frameworks
    120–1
    see also Knowledge and Skills Framework
APEL (Accredited for Prior Experiential
    Learning) 121
appraisal
    context and background 1
    defined 1, *2*
    terminology 3, *13–14*
appraisal action plans 45, 47–8, 110–11
    documentation 47, 105–7
    failures to achieve 52
    and half-year reviews 6, 52
    see also personal development plans
    (PDPs); professional development
    activities
appraisal forms 35, 104–7
    appraisee completion times 35
    completion problems 51–2
    and confidentiality 107
    formats 44
    general procedures 37, 106
    good practice guidelines 105–7
    see also appraisal action plans
appraisal meetings
    appraisee preparation techniques 35–9
    appraiser preparation and information
    needs 41–3, 43–4

dealing with hostile appraisees 123–4
dealing with underperforming
    appraisees 106–7, 110–11, 127–8
discussion issues 51–5, 110
general procedures and timescales
    36–7, *42*, 43–5
and non-participation 54, *172*
problems and pitfalls 45–7, 51–5
progress reviews *43*, 47, 110
session format and structure 44
session rules and objectives 45, 47–8,
    52, 54
setting performance targets 110–11
tips and techniques 44–5
see also appraisal schemes;
    communication skills; data from
    appraisals; feedback
appraisal schemes
    aims and objectives 3–4, 164
    and day-to-day supervision 41
    funding 167–8, *172*
    key success factors 8
    links with personal development plans
    (PDPs) 14–15, 18, 120–1, 122,
    125–6, 131–44
    management and administration needs
    171–4
    'marketing' and promotion 96
    NHS implementation rates 8
    NHS requirements 1, 145–6
    organisation (PCO) implementation
    considerations 6–8, 167–74
    and parallel objectives 7, 120–1
    systems for monitoring complaints *170*
    uses for collected data 8, 35
    see also appraisal meetings; evaluation of
    appraisal schemes; training appraisers
appraisee
    giving feedback on schemes 109,
    148–52
    health problems 103
    preparation tips for appraisals 35–9
    progress and learning outcomes 10–11
    underperformance 106–7

appraisers 41–55
    contracts and employment terms *170*,
        185–7
    and independent contractors 1, 52
    'job description' templates 175–7
    key skills *49*, *58*
    leadership skills 114–17
    as line manager 1, 52–3
    performance monitoring frameworks
        57–9, 60–117
    personal qualities *36*, 49–50
    relationship to appraisee 52
    role differentiation 50–1
    support and mentoring arrangements
        54, 168, *173*
    see also training appraisers
assertiveness 31–2
assessment
    defined *2*, *13*
    examinations used as evidence of
        competency 21
    see also feedback
audiotapes, as portfolio evidence *17*, 22
audit
    defined 19
    five stages 19–20

Belbin's self-perception inventory
    112–13
body language, in effective communication
    63

career counselling *132*
career reviews 131–44
    developing goals and aspirations
        139–41
    frameworks and plans *141–3*
    information sources *132*
    job evaluation and profiles 132–4
    and personal development plans (PDPs)
        135
    self-assessment of skills *138–9*
    see also personal development plans
careers guidance *132*
case note analysis 20
case studies
    and confidentiality 18
    as portfolio evidence *17*
change management 84–5
clinical governance, key principles 9

clinical supervisors 51
coaches 50, *51*
codes of conduct *see* Professional Code of
    Conduct (NMC 2002)
COGPED (Committee of General Practice
    Education Directors)
    recommendations 7
commercial training bodies 167
Committee of General Practice Education
    Directors (COGPED)
    recommendations 7
communication skills 60–76
    active listening 64
    and conflicts of interest 47, 52–3,
        74–6
    creating rapport 65–6
    and feedback 53, 70–4
    general tips *62*, *64*
    and the JoHari model 66–9
    language and meaning 62–4
    listening v. talking 49
    open-ended questions 65
    self-assessment 60–1
    trust and good relationships 69–70
competence 59, 119
    of appraisee 18, 103, 106–7
    of appraiser 49, 57–9, 60, 88, 93,
        96–7, 100, 102, 105, 109,
        119–28
    providing evidence and documentation
        57–9, 119–28
    and under performance 103, 109–10
complaints
    from appraisees *170*
    see also patient complaints
confidentiality
    and patient risk 103, 106–7
    in portfolio case studies 18
    within appraisals 42, 47, 107
conflict management 6, 53–4, 74–6,
    123–4
conflicts of interest 47, 52–3
continuing professional development (CPD)
    14–18
    links with GMS contracts/PMS practice
        arrangements 18
contracts *170*
    and general medical services (GMS)
        contract 11, 18
    for independent contractors 183–5

Council for the Regulation of Healthcare
    Professions 10
counsellors 50, *51*
criteria-based audit 20
criticism handling 53
    see also conflicts of interest; feedback

data from appraisals 47, 105–7
    completion times 106
    and confidentiality 107
    see also appraisal forms
Deaneries
    COGPED recommendations for roles and
        responsibilities 7
    Kent, Surrey and Sussex (KSS) Deanery
        vii–viii, 7
    training provisions 9
    Welsh GP appraisal scheme 9
    West Midlands Deanery evaluation
        systems/toolkits 157–8, *159–62,*
        171–4
definitions 50–1
    appraisal 1, *2*
    assessment 2
    audit 19
    competence 59
    evaluation 2–3
    mentoring 143
360 degree feedback 98, *127*
development needs review (DNR) *see*
        appraisal meetings; appraisal
        schemes
diaries and learning journals 16, 29
doctor's appraisal schemes
    and standards of practice 18
    see also appraisal schemes
documentation as evidence
    of appraiser competency 123–8
    and the 'stages of evidence cycle'
        119–22, 123–8
    see also Knowledge and Skills
        Framework; learning journals;
        portfolios
duplication 7
    using university frameworks for
        documenting prior learning 120–1

educational needs *see* learning needs
    assessment
educational strategies, and appraisals *173*

employment contracts *see* contracts
equal opportunities 100–1
    promotion through appraisals 99–101
evaluation, defined 2–3
evaluation of appraisal schemes 7–8, 57–8,
        145–64
    appraisee feedback 109, 148–52
    appraiser reviews 154–6, *156*
    the 'evaluation cycle' 146–7
    group-based schemes 153–5
    identifying importance of components
        147
    patient feedback 163
    and peer reviews 156–7
    and quality assurance 8–9
    quantitative measures 150, *162*
    using PDPs as evaluation tool 152–3
    West Midlands Deanery appraisal
        evaluation toolkit *159–62*
    workshop generated proposals *162*
    see also feedback
'evidence' of PDP/CPD *see* Knowledge and
        Skills Framework; portfolios
expert patient programme 21
external audits 20

feedback 70–4
    and 'criticism' 53
    360 degree model 98, *127*
    from appraisees 109, 148–52, *172*
    and the JoHari model 66–9
    key considerations 73
    and quality improvement initiatives 98
    see also evaluation of appraisal schemes
A First Class Service (DoH 1998) 1
force-field analysis, for work situation
        appraisals 80–2

gap analysis, for work situation appraisals
        83
general medical services (GMS) contract
    education/training/appraisal indicators
        11
    and professional development plans 18
GMS contract *see* general medical services
        (GMS) contract
Good Medical Practice (GMC) 9, 105, 109–10
GP's
    appraisal requirements 1, 9
    appraiser skills and competencies 49

PCT's appraisal responsibilities 9
training in appraisal management 9, 49
unacceptable standards of performance 109–10
group-based evaluation techniques 153–5

half-year reviews 6, 52
Healthcare Commission 163
health problems, and risk management 103
health and safety promotion skills 87–91
hospital consultants, appraisal requirements 1
hostility to appraisals 6, 53–4, 74–6, 123–4

Improving Working Lives (IWL) assessments, on appraisal scheme take-up 8
individual performance reviews (IPRs) *see* appraisal meetings; appraisal schemes
information sources 6–7
    Committee of General Practice Education Directors (COGPED) 6–7
    websites 6, 21, 98, 107, 188
    see also Deaneries; Nursing and Midwifery Council (NMC)
interpersonal assessments
    and team working 112–13
    see also peer appraisal; peer review of appraiser performance

jargon 62
job evaluations 133–4
    motivational factors and career fulfilment 134–5
JoHari models 66–9

Kent, Surrey and Sussex (KSS) Deanery vii–viii, 7
Kirkpatrick's hierarchy 2–3, *147*, 149, 159, 164
Knowledge and Skills Framework (KSF) 57–9, *58*
    background 57–8
    for developing communication effectiveness 58–76
    for developing leadership skills 114–17
    for enabling effective service delivery 87–117

for enabling professional/personal development 76–85
for enabling service development 92–6
for job evaluations 134
for learning needs assessment 108–11
and the management of appraisal processes 104–8
for promoting equal opportunities and rights 99–101
for promoting partnership and team working 111–13
for promoting quality improvement 96–9
for self-care and peer support 101–4
Knowles, MS 93
KSF tools *see* Knowledge and Skills Framework
KSS Deanery *see* Kent, Surrey and Sussex Deanery (KSS)

leadership skills 114–17
    promotion through appraisals 114–15
learning inventories 79–80
learning journals 16, 29
learning needs assessment 108–11, *152–3*
learning skills, and reflective practice 93
learning styles 24
Likert scales 151
listening skills 49, 64

maintaining confidentiality 107
mentoring, defined 143
mentors 50, *51*
    and career development 143–4
    see also shadowing
monitoring processes *see* evaluation of appraisal schemes
6 monthly reviews 6, 52
motivational skills 116

NHS Education for Scotland (NES), and GP appraisal schemes 9
NHS Knowledge and Skills Framework *see* Knowledge and Skills Framework
NHS Modernisation Agency's Leadership Centre, and 360 degree assessment process 98
NHS organisational changes, and need for half-year reviews 6
non-participation 54, *172*

North Stoke Teaching Primary Care Trust, employee appraisal scheme 4
Northern Ireland, Local Health and Social Care Groups GP appraisal schemes 9
Nursing and Midwifery Council (NMC), appraisal and portfolio requirements 1, 14–15

objectives in appraisal agreements see appraisal action plans
organisational (PCO) objectives
    and appraisal 4–6
    educational strategies 173
    initial support systems and protocols 169, 170
    resource needs 167–8
    support through quality assurance frameworks 171–4

partnership working 111–13
patient case studies
    and confidentiality 18
    as portfolio evidence 17
patient complaints
    and portfolios 21
    use as quantitative appraisal evaluation tool 150
patient safety
    and appraisee health problems 103
    and appraisee underperformance 107
patient satisfaction surveys, as portfolio evidence 17, 21
PCO (primary care organisation) objectives see organisational (PCO) objectives
PDPs see personal development plans
peer appraisal 1, 49
    and feelings of intimidation 54
peer review of appraiser performance 20, 156–8
performance management 3–4, 14
    and integration of appraisal schemes 5–6, 5
    see also competence; professional regulation; standards of practice
performance standards see standards of practice
performance targets for appraisees see appraisal action plans

personal development plans (PDPs) 14–16
    analysis tools and templates 79–83, 178–81
    and career development 131, 135
    evaluation tools 152–3, 173
    job evaluation 133–4
    quality 182–4
    personal motivation and work values 134–5
    use as appraisal scheme evaluation tools 152–3
personal learning inventory 79–80
personal medical services (PMS) practice arrangements
    appraisal requirements 1
    and professional development plans 18
portfolios
    and doctors revalidation 10
    nurses 1, 14–15
    preparation considerations 16–17
    professional v. organisational requirements 7, 18
    tools and techniques 19–24
    types of material/evidence 16, 17, 19–24
    and use of audit 19–21
post-registration education and practice standards (PREP) 15
postgraduate awards, using university frameworks for documenting prior learning 120–1
preceptors 51
PREP (post-registration education and practice standards) 15
preparation techniques for appraisals 35–9
prior learning accreditation 121
Professional Code of Conduct (NMC 2002) 14, 18
professional development activities
    healthcare context 78
    preparations for appraisals 35–9
    self-assessment of knowledge base 77–8
    stress management 29–34, 89–90
    time management 25–9
    see also appraisers; career reviews; competence; personal development plans; portfolios
professional regulation
    and the Council for the Regulation of Healthcare Professions 10

CPD/PDP and PMS/GMS arrangements 18
and duplication 7
Nursing and Midwifery Council (NMC) 1, 14–15
and post-registration education and practice standards (PREP) 15
and revalidation 9–10
profiling health needs 23
progress reviews, within appraisal schemes 43
psychometric measurements, and team working 112
public health, use of local needs profiles in portfolios 23

qualitative evaluation analysis techniques 150–2
quality assurance 8–9
toolkits and frameworks for appraisals 171–4
quality improvement 97–8
Deming's 14 points 98
promotion through the appraisal process 96–9
quantitative evaluation measures 150
questionnaires, for patient satisfaction surveys 21

rating scales, use in appraisal scheme evaluations 151–2
record keeping see data from appraisals; documentation as evidence
reflective practices
encouraging skill development through staff appraisals 92–6
learning logs 16, 29
reading and recording articles 22
see also Knowledge and Skills Framework (KSF); portfolios
revalidation 9–10, 14
and appraisee underperformance 107
comparisons with appraisal 10
risk assessments
appraisee performance problems and patient safety 103, 107
use in personal development portfolios 22–3
risk management skills 87–91
round robin evaluations 154

Royal College of General Practitioners' (RCGP), quality awards 21

safety and security arrangement audits 87–91
satisfaction surveys
patient feedback 17, 21
see also evaluation of appraisal schemes
Schein, E 134
Scotland, NES and GP appraisal schemes 9
self-care and health 101–3
self-esteem 34, 53, 135
service development
encouraging reflective practice through staff appraisals 92–6
identification of issues for use in portfolios 23–4, 121
and leadership 114–17
sexual attraction 53
shadowing 113
significant event audits 20–1, 99
use in stress management 30
snowball reviews 154–5
social support networks 32–3
staff appraisals see appraisal meetings; appraisal schemes
staff attitudes, to appraisal scheme implementation 6
staff health
appraisee problems and patient risk management 103
self-care 101–3
staff security 87–91
staff support services 89
'stages of evidence cycle' 119–22
use in case studies 123–8
standards of practice
doctors 18
levels of performance 109–10
and underperformance 103, 106–7, 109–10
see also Professional Code of Conduct (NMC 2002); professional regulation
stress management
techniques and preventative strategies 29–34, 89–90
see also self-care and health
summative evaluations 145–6
support networks 32–3
SWOT analysis 94–5

teaching activities, documenting
        experiences/jobs 125–6
team working 111–13
time management
    and appraisals 117
    and PDPs 25
    techniques 25–9
timetables for appraisals 36–7, *42*, 43–5,
        55, 117
training appraisers 6–7, 167–8, *171–3*
    in documentation skills 119–28
    in effective communication skills 9,
        58–76
    to enable effective service delivery
        87–117
    to enable professional/personal
        development 3–4, 76–85
    to enable service development 92–6
    in leadership skills 114–17
    in learning needs assessment 108–11,
        152–3
    in management of appraisal processes
        104–8
    in partnership and team working
        111–13
    in promoting equal opportunities and
        rights 99–101
    in quality improvement 96–9
    in self-care and peer support 101–4
    in support needs and resources 167–8,
        173

use of video records 157–8
    see also competence
trust issues 69–70

video records
    as portfolio evidence 16, 22
    use in evaluation of appraiser
        performance 157–8

waiting time audits, use in personal
        development portfolios 22
Wales, and GP appraisal schemes 9
websites 6, 188
    on appraisal system development 6
    NHS leadership qualities 98
    Nursing and Midwifery Council (NMC)
        1
    on patient satisfaction surveys 21
    revalidation and appraisals 107
West Midlands Deanery
    evaluation of appraisals 157–62
    quality assurance toolkit for appraisals
        171–4
workforce attitudes to appraisal schemes 6
workplace security 89–91
workshops
    for developing/evaluating appraisal
        schemes 169, *172*, 174
    as support for appraisers 168
WWP (What Went Well, Why, Plan) reviews
        155